THE
AYURVEDA
BIBLE

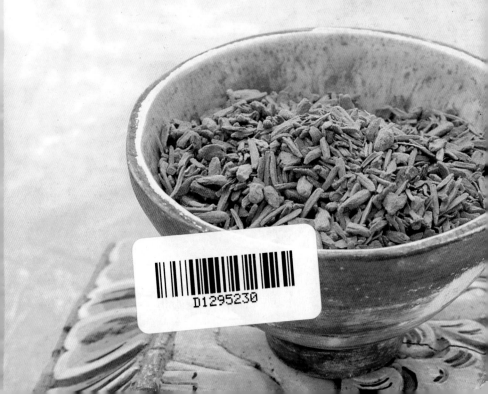

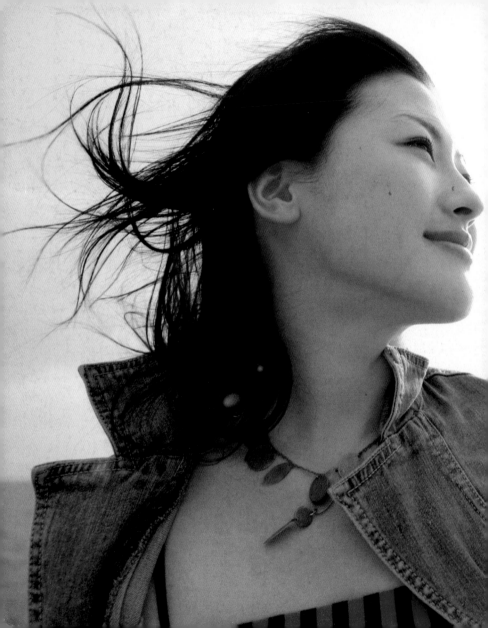

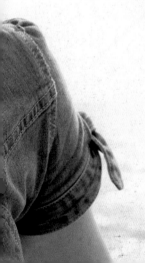

THE
AYURVEDA
BIBLE

THE DEFINITIVE GUIDE TO AYURVEDIC HEALING

ANNE MCINTYRE

FIREFLY BOOKS

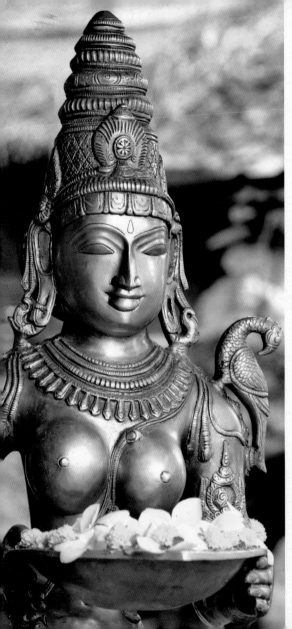

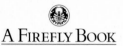

A FIREFLY BOOK

Published by Firefly Books Ltd. 2012

Copyright © Octopus Publishing Group Ltd. 2012
Text copyright © Anne McIntyre 2012

First printing

Publisher Cataloging-in-Publication Data (U.S.)

McIntyre, Anne.
   The ayurveda bible : the definitive guide to ayurvedic healing / Anne McIntyre.
[400] p. : col. ill., col. photos. ; cm.
Includes index.
Summary: Comprehensive guide explores the Indian healing system of ayurveda, from its origins in ancient Vedic scriptures to ayurveda as practiced today. Includes how to work towards optimum health through diet, lifestyle, exercise and spiritual practices, according to individual dosha or constitution type, and detailed recommendations for the holistic treatment of common ailments, with herbs, food, massage and meditation.
ISBN-13: 9781770850446 (pbk.)
1. Medicine, Ayurvedic. I. Title.
615.53 dc23   R606.M3568 2012

Library and Archives Canada Cataloguing in Publication

McIntyre, Anne
   The Ayurveda bible : the definitive guide to Ayurvedic healing / Anne McIntyre.
Includes index.
ISBN 978-1-77085-044-6
   1. Medicine, Ayurvedic. I. Title.
R606.M35 2012   615.5'38   C2011-906526-6

Published in the United States by
Firefly Books (U.S.) Inc.
P.O. Box 1338, Ellicott Station
Buffalo, New York 14205

Published in Canada by
Firefly Books Ltd.
66 Leek Crescent
Richmond Hill, Ontario L4B 1H1

Printed in China

Developed and produced by Godsfield, a division of Octopus Publishing Group Ltd, Endeavour House
189 Shaftesbury Avenue, London WC2H 8JY

Contents

Introduction

This book is an easy-to-follow and practical introduction to Ayurveda, the traditional natural healing system of India. Ayurveda is an ancient philosophy based on a deep understanding of eternal truths about the human body, mind and spirit which is rapidly growing in popularity in the West. It offers us advice about how to keep ourselves healthy and to rebalance us when we become unwell. This book is ideal for anyone wanting to discover how Ayurveda can help them in their own life as well as for practitioners wishing to increase their healing repertoire.

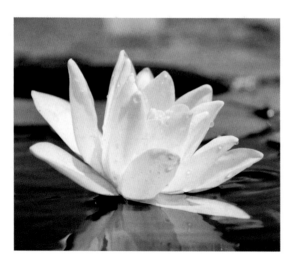

The lotus is the national flower of India and its petals represent the eight branches of Ayurveda.

The first part of this book, 'Understanding Ayurveda', defines Ayurveda and describes its history, placing it in the wider context of the development of medical philosophy in the East and its influence on that of medicine in the West. Ayurveda has survived through millennia until now largely as an unbroken tradition; two of its greatest values are its timelessness and its application to every facet of daily living today, just as it was relevant all those centuries ago. This book goes on to explain the philosophy and cosmology of Ayurveda, and explores its fundamental principles in detail. It describes and explains the basic tenets of Ayurvedic theory which are important to understand before you go on to consider treatment. It includes the five elements, the three *doshas* and their subtypes, the seven *dhatus*,

These traditional Ayurveda recipes have been written on palm leaves.

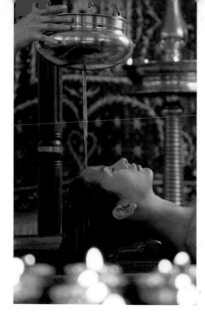

Shirodhara is one of the best Ayurvedic treatments to calm the mind.

the *malas*, the 20 attributes, and the *srotas*.

The second part of the book, 'Maintaining health and well-being', describes the three *gunas*, the prime energies of the universe that primarily affect the mind and advises a way of life to enhance inner peace and joy. It explains how to assess your Ayurvedic constitution, the balance of your three *doshas*, and includes a questionnaire. It goes on to explain the vital role of *Agni*, the digestive fire, in health and the prevention of disease and explains how the six tastes of foods and herbs can be used as tools for prevention as well as treatment.

Part 3, 'Ayurvedic diagnosis and treatment', looks firstly at the causes and stages of disease from an Ayurvedic perspective, then at the art of diagnosis in all its forms, including tongue and pulse diagnosis. It explores the range of treatments you can use at home to balance the *doshas* and treat the *dhatus*, and the importance of detoxification to restore health to body and mind.

Lastly, part 4, 'Tools of Ayurvedic treatment', comprises a comprehensive directory of 50 of the most commonly used and available Ayurvedic herbs, followed by details of well-known Ayurvedic preparations and formulae. It describes *Panchakarma*, the deep and thorough detoxification

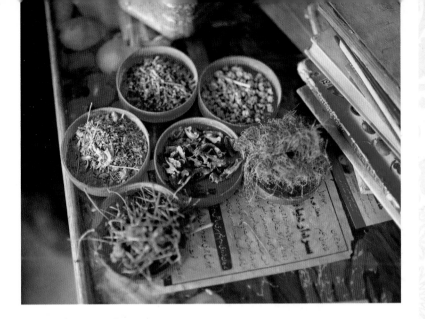

Herbs are used both fresh and dried in a wide range of different formulations.

practices of Ayurveda, and finishes with a discussion of *Rasayana*, the Ayurvedic science of rejuvenation.

I have used Ayurveda in my own practice as a herbalist for 20 years or so. As my knowledge of Ayurveda has increased I have found it an invaluable tool for helping myself and others understand how to prevent and treat health problems.

The Ayurvedic approach emphasizes the importance of addressing the roots of health and disease rather than the thousands of disease symptoms which arise from these roots. It is an approach that is simple without being simplistic and can be grasped by any of us wanting to maximize our healing potential through an understanding of ourselves and the universe around us.

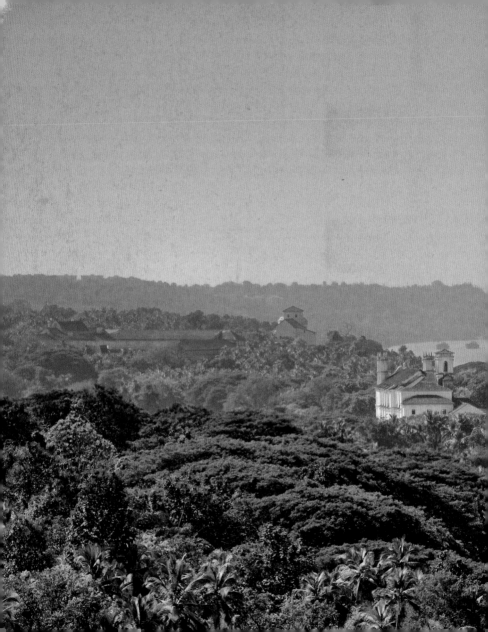

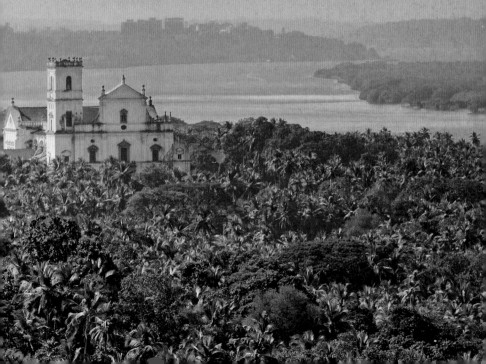

PART 1
UNDERSTANDING AYURVEDA

The first part of the book explores the long history of Ayurveda and how the way of life advocated by the great wisdom of this ancient system of knowledge can help you achieve health and longevity through a union of physical, emotional and spiritual balance. It explains the basic philosophy of Ayurveda, and then explores its fundamental principles in detail.

Chapter 1: The history and philosophy of Ayurveda

The traditional healing system of India, Ayurveda is believed to be the oldest-surviving complete medical system in the world. As a more global view of medicine, philosophy and spirituality develops, Ayurveda's popularity in the West is soaring today.

Ayurveda is actually much more than a system of medicine; it embraces medical science, philosophy, psychology, alchemy and spiritual understanding, as well as astrology and astronomy. Its tools include lifestyle guidance, herbal medicine, nutrition, detoxification, massage and other body work, plus spiritual practices. It is based on the accumulated knowledge and understanding of millennia and yet it is very up to date, offering practical and effective treatment for many modern disorders that affect both mind and body. Clinical trials are being carried out at major Ayurvedic institutions as the search continues for treatments that are safe and effective. This means that ancient wisdom that has stood the test of time for countless generations is increasingly being verified by modern research.

Ayurveda embraces massage and other body work as well as spiritual practices.

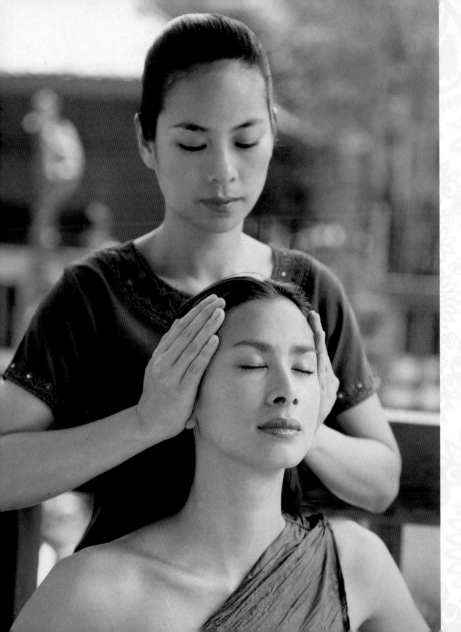

A little history

The ancient philosophy of Ayurveda is based on a deep understanding of eternal truths about the human body, mind and spirit. There has been much speculation about its true origins, which may go back 5,000 years or more.

Early literature preserved by Buddhist monks provides evidence that Ayurveda evolved as a medical and philosophical tradition from the deep wisdom of spiritually enlightened prophets or seers known as *Rishis*, who lived in the far reaches of the Himalayas in northern India. Their wisdom – encompassing Ayurveda, yoga and meditation – was transmitted orally from teacher to disciple and was eventually set down in Sanskrit poetry known as the Vedas (more specifically, the Rig Veda and the Atharva Veda). These writings distilled the prevailing historical, religious, philosophical and medical knowledge at the time, and form the foundations of Indian culture and religion, particularly Hinduism, from which the whole of Indian culture derived and diversified.

Early physicians

Around 800 BCE the first Ayurvedic medical school was founded by a famous physician called Punarvasu Atreya. Atreya and his pupils recorded medical knowledge in treatises that would in turn influence Charaka, a scholar who lived and taught around 700 BCE. His writings, the Charaka Samhita, describe 1,500 plants, identifying 350 as valuable medicines. This major text is still

THE EIGHT BRANCHES OF AYURVEDA

The symbol of Ayurveda is the beautiful lotus flower, with its eight petals representing the eight branches of Ayurveda as described in the Atharva Veda, which are:

- *Kayachikitsa* – internal medicine
- *Salya tantra* – surgery
- *Salakya tantra* – treatment of the ears, nose, throat, eyes and teeth
- *Agada tantra* – toxicology, the study of poisons
- *Bhuta vidya* – psychiatry, the treatment of mental disease
- *Bala tantra* – gynaecology, obstetrics and paediatrics
- *Rasayana tantra* – the science of rejuvenation
- *Vajikarana tantra* – aphrodisiacs to increase potency and life.

considered the main authority of Ayurveda and is constantly referred to in both the teaching and practice of Ayurveda today.

The second major work was the Susruta Samhita, written a century later, which forms the basis of modern surgery and is consulted to this day. The Astanga Hridayam is a more concise compilation of earlier texts that dates from about a thousand years ago.

Ayurvedic influences

Ayurveda has had a strong influence on many systems of medicine, from ancient Greek medicine in the West to

Traditional Chinese Medicine in the East. All forms of philosophy of India (including that of the Jains and Sikhs) have the same basic principles, which are in harmony with the spiritual background of Ayurveda. The Chinese, Tibetan and Islamic (Unani Tibb) systems of medicine are also thought to have their roots in Ayurveda.

The Buddha, who was born around 550 BCE, was a follower of Ayurveda, and so the spread of Buddhism by monks into Tibet, China, Mongolia, Korea and Sri Lanka in the following centuries was accompanied by increased practice of Ayurveda. The ancient civilizations were linked to one another by trade routes and wars. Arab traders spread knowledge of Indian plants in their Materia Medicas, and this knowledge was passed on to the ancient Greeks and Romans, whose philosophies and practices were eventually to form the basis of European medicine.

Ayurveda has survived largely as an unbroken oral tradition until the present day, despite a number of setbacks. Two of its greatest values are its timelessness and its application to every facet of daily living today, just as it applied all those centuries ago.

Following the rise of the Mogul empire in the 16th century, the dominance of Unani Tibb (Islamic) medicine led to the partial repression of Ayurveda in India. In the 19th century the British dismissed it as nothing more than native superstition and in 1833 closed all Ayurvedic schools and banned the practice of Ayurveda. Great centres of Indian learning thus fell apart, and Ayurvedic knowledge retreated into the villages and temples.

Ayurveda's renaissance

At the start of the 20th century, however, some Indian physicians and enlightened Englishmen began to re-evaluate Ayurveda, and by the time India had become independent in 1947 it had regained its reputation as a valid healing system. Today Ayurveda flourishes in India alongside Unani Tibb and Western allopathic (conventional) medicine and is actively encouraged by the Indian government as an inexpensive alternative to Western drugs.

In recent years Ayurveda has increasingly attracted attention from medical scientists in Japan and the West, and the World Health Organization has resolved to promote its practice in developing countries. In the West its popularity grows daily, as more and more people recognize its immense value – not only in the prevention and treatment of disease, but for its comprehensive recipe for a better, healthier way of life that addresses all facets of our existence: mind, body and spirit.

Ayurveda has a comprehensive recipe for a better, healthier way of life.

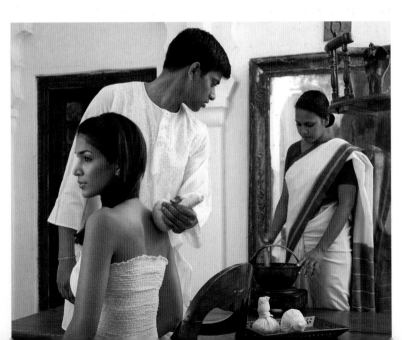

Ayurvedic philosophy

The term Ayurveda is derived from the Sanskrit *ayur*, meaning 'life' or 'longevity', and *veda*, meaning 'knowledge', 'wisdom' or 'spiritual science'; so Ayurveda is a complete body of knowledge and profound wisdom about how to live to achieve health (*Swasthya*) and longevity through a union of physical, emotional and spiritual balance in order to achieve *Moksha* (enlightenment).

According to Ayurveda there is a fundamental truth, a state of pure consciousness beyond word and thought, in which there is bliss, love, compassion and liberation. This is *Moksha*, or enlightenment, and to reach it is the goal of life. Without *Moksha* as our ultimate goal, life is essentially a state of suffering caused by the ego, which sets in motion a stream of *Karma*, or action and reaction (cause and effect), tying us to the process of rebirth and the experience of repeated sorrow.

At the heart of Ayurveda lies the understanding that everything is One – meaning that everything exists in relation, not in isolation. Body affects mind, and vice versa; feelings and thoughts have physical effects, just as disorders of the body affect our psychological state.

Cosmic principles

Ayurveda and yoga share a special understanding of cosmic evolution that came from *Sankhya*'s philosophy of creation and manifestation. *Sankhya* is one of the six classical schools of Indian philosophy, as devised and expounded by the great seer

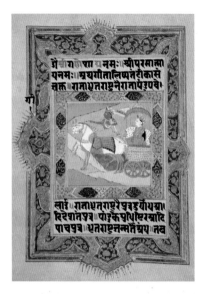

The Bhagavad Gita makes reference to Kapila, the great seer who is said to have devised Sankhya philosophy.

Kapila, who is mentioned in Vedic literature, from the Rig Veda to the Bhagavad Gita.

Sankhya means 'the system of enumerology' because it has categorized its theory of evolution into 24 cosmic principles (*Tattvas*), from the unmanifest realm of pure existence to the material, manifest world. Although they seem to be sequential, in fact they all occur simultaneously. *Purusha*, or pure consciousness, is listed as the 25th principle; it is described here first because it forms the foundation of the following 24 principles and transcends them all.

Purusha (pure consciousness)

According to *Sankhya*, the origin of all aspects of existence is pure consciousness – supreme intelligence that is all-pervading, beyond time and space, with no qualities, no form, no beginning and no end – known as *Purusha*. *Purusha* is pure passive awareness, and within us it is the silent observer, the indwelling being or 'Atman', the inner or higher self. Within this subtle state of stillness arises a desire to experience itself, which causes the manifestation of the primordial physical energy

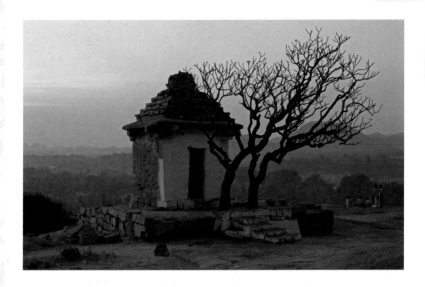

According to Ayurveda everything that exists in the macrocosm has its counterpart in the microcosm of our inner universe.

known as *Prakruti*, and this is the origin of the manifested world. *Purusha* is regarded as masculine energy, while *Prakruti* is the female seed holding the potential of everything in creation. Together they unite to create movement that causes the 'dance of creation' to begin.

1 *Prakruti* (primordial nature)

Prakruti literally means 'the first power of action', for it is the creative force behind everything in the universe. The womb of creation, *Prakruti* is also called *Pradhana* (meaning first substance), as it is the unmanifest essence of all substance in the universe, both gross and subtle. Ayurveda does not separate the external from the inner world.

Everything that exists in the macrocosm has its counterpart in the microcosm of the inner universe of the human being.

2 *Mahat* (cosmic intelligence)

Prakruti gives rise to cosmic consciousness, known as *Mahat*, which is the universal or cosmic intelligence underlying everything in creation.

Mahat literally means 'the great', for it is the divine mind whose intelligence creates the great laws and principles that govern life. It is the archetypal forms behind the manifest world.

Within the individual, *Mahat* becomes *Buddhi*, our inner wisdom – the part of us that maintains objectivity, unaffected by the demands of daily life or by *Ahamkara*, the sense of 'I-ness'. *Buddhi* gives us our innate intelligence, which enables us to perceive the truth, know right from wrong, real from unreal and the eternal from the transient.

3 *Ahamkara* (ego)

Ahamkara literally means 'the I-maker', for the ego is in fact a process, not an intrinsic reality. This process involves identification with different aspects of the created world, such as thinking 'I am cold' in winter and identifying with this feeling. So *Ahamkara* is a series of divisive thoughts, not a separate entity, despite the fact that we conceive it as a consistent self with which we identify. It is the aspect of ourselves that creates the illusion of separateness from cosmic consciousness, and thus causes so much suffering.

4 *Manas* (conditional mind)

Manas means 'the formulating principle', from the root *man*, to form. It connects us to the outer world through the senses. *Manas* is the mind as it experiences and registers perceptions and sensations received through the five senses, and then identifies and conceptualizes ideas and emotions. It is mental functioning.

5–9 The five *Tanmatras*

The five *Tanmatras* are the 'primal measures' illustrating the fivefold energy structure of the cosmos, which pervades everything in creation. They are the five senses of sound, touch, sight, taste and smell that enable us to connect the five sense organs with objects of experience. They are the subtle forms of the five elements of ether, air, fire, water and earth, before their differentiation becomes manifest in the material world. They are:

- *Shabda Tanmatra* – sound
- *Sparsha Tanmatra* – touch
- *Rupa Tanmatra* – sight
- *Rasa Tanmatra* – taste
- *Gandha Tanmatra* – smell.

10–14 *Pancha Jnanendriyani* (the five sense organs)

It is the five sense organs that enable us to experience the outer world, and these connect to the five elements as follows:

- Ears, the sense organ of sound, to the element of ether
- Skin, the sense organ of touch, to the element of air
- Eyes, the sense organ of sight, to the element of fire
- Tongue, the sense organ of taste, to the element of water
- Nose, the sense organ of smell, to the element of earth.

These sense organs are receptive only, not expressive. Their activity occurs through the corresponding organs of action. Subtle or inner forms of these organs also exist beyond the limitations of the physical body, and their action gives us extrasensory perception, or ESP.

15–19 *Pancha Karmendriyani* (the five organs of action)

These physical structures enable us to communicate and manifest ourselves, and correspond to the five sense organs and the five elements. They are expressive, not receptive:

- Mouth (expression), corresponding to ether and sound

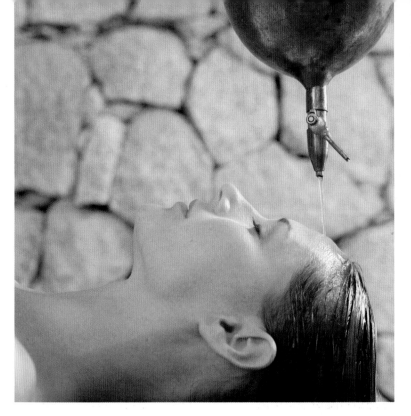

- Hands (grasping), corresponding to air and touch
- Feet (motion), corresponding to fire and sight
- Penis (vagina), corresponding to water and taste
- Anus (elimination), corresponding to earth and smell.

Skin is one of the five sense organs. It is the organ of touch, connected to the element of air.

20–24 *Pancha Mahabhuta* (the five great elements)

Cosmic energy manifests in the five elements, which are the basis of all matter and apply to all manifestation, including the mind – namely, ether, air, fire, water and earth (see page 28). Going from the most subtle to the most gross, they represent the etheric, gaseous, radiant, liquid and solid aspects of matter respectively, which compose the outer world of experience, including the physical body.

The five elements manifest in the functioning of the five senses, and these in turn enable us to perceive and interact with the environment in which we live. Ether, air, fire, water and earth correspond to hearing, touch, vision, taste and smell respectively.

The three *gunas*

Prakruti is composed of three prime qualities, or *gunas*: *Sattva*, *Rajas* and *Tamas*. They are more subtle than the five elements that arise through their activity. They also precede the *Tanmatras*.

• From *Sattva* arise the five sense organs
• From *Rajas* arise the five organs of action
• From *Tamas* arise the five elements.

Everything in the universe is a different combination of the three *gunas*. *Sattva* is the highest quality of light, harmony, virtue, happiness, clarity and intelligence; *Rajas* is the quality of movement, distraction, turbulence and activity; while *Tamas* is the quality of dullness, darkness, decay, inertia and rest to enable regeneration. They represent the potential for differentiation in *Prakruti*, the causal factors of creation, while the five senses (*Tanmatras*) are the subtle factors and the five elements are the gross effects.

Under the predominance of *Tamas*, the five elements evolve with diversification according to the three *gunas*:
• Ether comes from *Sattva*
• Fire comes from *Rajas*
• Earth comes from *Tamas*
• Air is composed of *Sattva* and *Rajas* (lightness and movement)

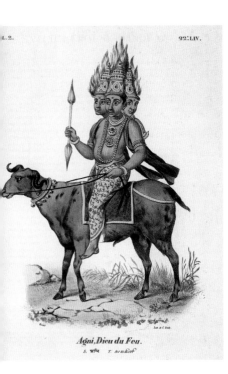

L. 2.   22?LIV.

Agni, Dieu du Feu.
S. आग्नि   T. நெருப்பு

Agni *is the two-headed god of fire from the* Rig Veda *who reveals the true nature of one's own self.*

The three *doshas*

The three *doshas*, or biological 'humours' that govern our constitution – *Vata*, *Pitta* and *Kapha* – arise primarily through *Rajas*, as they are kinds of mobile or vital energies, and they each have five different forms (see page 32).

The *doshas* provide the physiological structure for the interplay of the organs and elements that become the physical body. The five types of *Vata* allow for the coordination of the five sense organs and the five organs of action, meaning that sensory input can be responded to by action.

- Water has both *Rajas* and *Tamas* (movement and heaviness)
- Earth is pure *Tamas*.

The right balance of the three *gunas* is called 'pure *Sattva*', as it occurs through a predominance and refinement of *Sattva*.

The four goals of life

According to Vedic philosophy there are four rightful goals in life, and all human beings aspire to one or more of them: *Kama*

Ayurveda was recorded in Sanskrit poetry known as the Vedas *which are still important spiritual texts today.*

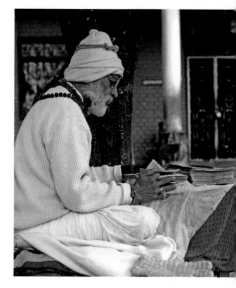

(enjoyment), *Artha* (prosperity), *Dharma* (career) and *Moksha* (enlightenment).

• *Kama*, meaning enjoyment, is our most basic goal. We all have a desire to be happy and avoid suffering, to enjoy the world of sensory experience and the satisfaction of emotional desires.

• *Artha* refers to the acquisition of wealth and possessions in the material world. We all need vital possessions like food, clothing and shelter in order to stay alive. This is the outer goal of the ego-principle (*Ahamkara*).

• *Dharma*, meaning career, refers to the attainment of status, as recognition of our abilities, gifts, skills or talents, so that we can fulfil our role in life. This is the inner goal of the ego-principle.

• *Moksha*, meaning enlightenment, bliss, spiritual liberation and recognition of our own true nature.

The fundamental purpose in life is *Moksha*, true inner knowledge and liberation from suffering to enable us to reach our full potential. It is the *Sattvic* goal of intelligence or reason (*Buddhi*), which is not really a goal, but our own true nature, which we can come to through awareness and surrender of the ego and its endless seeking of goals. The other three goals arise from *Rajas* and are outer or secondary; when they become ends in themselves, they give rise to attitudes, beliefs and behaviour that can predispose us to physical and mental imbalance and disease. *Kama* as a primary goal is said to lead to overindulgence and dissipation of vital energy; *Artha* can lead to greed and selfish acquisitiveness; *Dharma* can lead to the pursuit of fame, power and control. *Moksha* represents freedom from attachment to the first three goals and a state of inner peace and joy.

THE GOAL OF AYURVEDA

Through Sankhya philosophy we can understand the Ayurvedic perspective that the universe is a manifestation of *Purusha* (supreme intelligence), which evolves and expresses itself in matter (*Prakruti*), in order to explore all aspects of experience inherent within itself. In this way the universe exists to provide experience for consciousness. Ayurveda provides the path to bring us back to knowledge of the spirit, or *Purusha*. It opens our awareness and teaches us that we are not just the body; this is a tool or vehicle for the expression of consciousness. Through the array of tools offered to us by this amazing body of knowledge we have the chance to connect to our own true nature. Until we do this, we will be prone to the process of degeneration that is inherent in the manifest world. Thus we can see that the only real cure for dis-ease is knowledge of the Self.

Chapter 2: **The principles of Ayurveda**

Human beings are constantly interacting with the universe and its elements, and vice versa. We fill space, which gives us a place to live and function in all our myriad ways; we breathe the air, drink water, keep ourselves warm with heat and light, and consume food provided by the earth. As long as our relationship with the universe is healthy and wholesome, we can be in optimum health. According to Ayurveda, when this harmonious interaction breaks down it pre-disposes us to dysfunction and disease.

The five elements
Ayurveda states that everything in the universe is composed of energy, and this energy exists in five different states of density, giving rise to five elements (*Pancha Mahabhuta*), namely:
- Ether/space (*Akasha*)
- Air/motion (*Vayu*)
- Fire/radiant energy (*Teja*)
- Water/cohesive factor (*Jala*)
- Earth/mass (*Prithvi*)

These five elements are not to be interpreted literally, but rather as metaphors that help us to understand the universe. They represent five qualities of energy that we can recognize as we experience them daily in our physical, mental and emotional lives.

How the five elements were formed
According to Ayurveda, everything originally consisted of pure consciousness, non-material

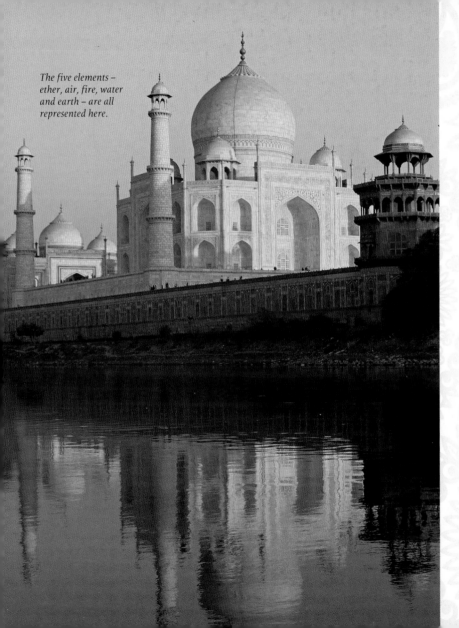

The five elements –
ether, air, fire, water
and earth – are all
represented here.

energy. From cosmic vibrations the most subtle element – ether – was formed. When it began to move it created the air element. Friction between moving elements gave rise to heat and the fire element. The fire melted and liquefied and created water, some of which in turn solidified, forming earth.

The human body is similarly composed of these five elements, and so it reflects the greater universe – it is a microcosm of the macrocosm. The five elements exist together everywhere in all things, constantly changing and interacting, in an infinite variety of proportions, and each of them has a range of different attributes.

Fire has the quality of heat and light and is the element that governs perception and transformation.

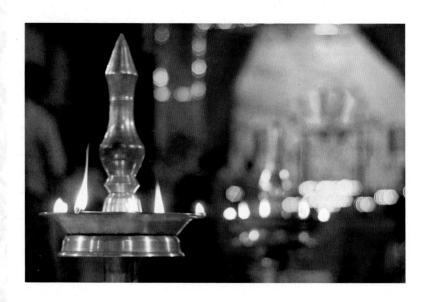

THE FIVE ELEMENTS AND THEIR ATTRIBUTES

- **Ether** means space that allows for the existence of everything, including communication between one part of the body and another – for instance, synaptic space, intracellular space, abdominal space – as well as self-expression.

- **Air** is gaseous and has airy qualities. It is light, clear, dry and dispersing. It governs all movement, direction and change, stirring all of creation into life. Air is present in the lungs and abdomen, for example, and its quality of movement can be seen in all movements in the body, particularly those of messages throughout the nervous system.

- **Fire** has the quality of light and heat, and it is dry and upward-moving. It governs perception and all transformation in the body. It is responsible for the temperature and colour of the body, for the lustre on the cheeks, the sheen of the hair, the light in the eyes.

- **Water** is liquidity or flowing motion, which gives cohesiveness and holds everything together. It is cool and downward-flowing and has no shape of its own. It is present in all the body's fluids, including blood, urine, stools, saliva and mucus.

- **Earth** is matter, solidity or stability. It is heavy and hard and gives the body form and substance. It is present in physical structure of the body: the organs, muscles and bones, teeth and tendons.

The *doshas*

As we have seen, there are three primary life forces or 'humours' derived from the five elements known as *doshas* – *Vata*, *Pitta* and *Kapha* – which are responsible for all functions in the body, both physical and psychological.

The *doshas* are created as follows:
• Ether and air create the air principle, **Vata**
• Fire and water yield the fire principle, **Pitta**
• Earth and water produce the water principle, **Kapha**.

Our constitution

We are all born with our own particular balance of *doshas*, which creates our constitution, and that remains unaltered throughout our lives. The predominant *dosha* (or *doshas*) determines our physique, our mental and emotional tendencies and our predisposition to certain health problems. We generally have a predominance of one or two of the *doshas*.

Our constitution (*Prakruti*) is largely determined when we are conceived and depends on our parents' constitutions, the balance of their *doshas* and their mental and emotional state at the time of conception, and of course their *Karma*. The characteristics of our dominant *dosha(s)* will be most apparent in our make-up, but naturally they are diluted by those of the other *doshas*.

To be alive and well, we need all three *doshas* and all five elements. When our *doshas* are in balance – that is, when they remain in the proportions that we were born with – they maintain our health and well-being; and when they are unbalanced we become unwell.

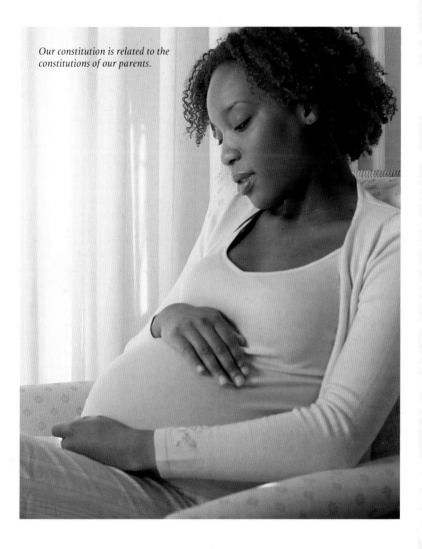

Our constitution is related to the constitutions of our parents.

Vata

A combination of ether and air, *Vata* is the principle of movement. The word *Vata* means 'wind', from the Sanskrit root *va*, meaning to blow, direct, move or command. *Vata* is our life force (*Prana*), derived primarily from the breath.

It is the energizing force for everything in body and mind, and this is reflected in the circulation of blood and lymph and every impulse of the nervous system. It is the motivating force behind the other two *doshas*, which are incapable of movement without it. For this reason, disturbances of *Vata* tend to have more far-reaching implications than those of the other two *doshas* and often affect the mind as well as the entire body.

In the body *Vata* controls all movement:
• Blinking of the eyes
• Movement of air in and out of the lungs

VATA QUALITIES	
• Dry	• Hard
• Cold	• Mobile
• Light	• Subtle
• Irregular	• Rough
• Sharp	• Clear

• Pulsations of the heart
• Movement of nerve impulses through the nervous system
• Movements involved with digestion and metabolism
• Elimination of wastes
• Circulation of blood and lymph
• Movement of nutrients into, and wastes out of, cells

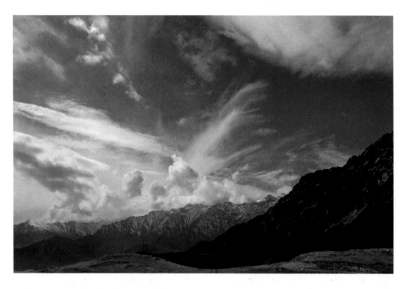

- Homoeostasis (balance) of the whole body.

Mentally and emotionally, *Vata* governs:
- Mental balance and well-being
- Movement of ideas in the mind
- Inspiration, creativity
- Spiritual aspiration
- Mental adaptability
- Comprehension
- Fear, insecurity, anxiety
- Vision and imagination.

Vata is a combination of the elements of ether and air. It is the principle of movement, like the wind.

The main sites of *Vata*

Vata is air contained in space (ether). It is found in the empty spaces in the body, like the heart, thorax, abdomen, pelvis, the pores of the bones, bone marrow, brain, bladder and the subtle channels of the nervous system. The lower abdomen is the site where *Vata* accumulates, and this includes the pelvis, urinary and reproductive tracts, bowel and lower back. The thighs and hips are the main site of musculoskeletal movement in the body, for which *Vata* is responsible. The ears and the skin – the organs of hearing and touch – are also governed by *Vata*. *Vata* is excreted from the body via gas and through muscular or nervous energy.

Vata's task in the body is to ensure there is enough space for the air to move in and sufficient movement in that space. Air can move freely through the body only when its paths are free of obstacles. Spasm and phlegm, for example, can obstruct the flow of air through the lungs, as in asthma. If there is too much space and insufficient movement it can cause stasis, or inactivity, as in emphysema and constipation.

Vata-predominant people tend to have narrow frames and a slight build.

Vata people

Like the wind, *Vata*-predominant people are changeable, and irregularity will feature strongly in their physical and emotional make-up. They may be very tall or very short, with a narrow or irregular frame and a slight build. They may have crooked teeth or irregular eyes (perhaps one being larger than the other) or their nose may not be straight. Their weight can change

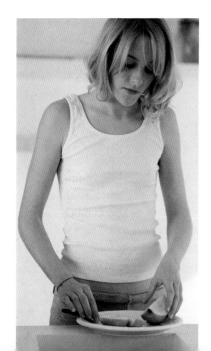

quickly and, when unhappy or stressed, they can lose weight easily. Some find it impossible to put on weight, while others become overweight from stress, digestive problems and eating badly. They tend to have prominent bones and joints that often crack. Their appetite is variable: sometimes they are ravenous, while at other times they have no appetite at all. As a result they tend to eat irregularly as they find it hard to be still. However, if they do not eat regularly, they become hypoglycaemic and can easily feel faint or weak and then even more anxious.

Vata-predominant people tend to feel the cold and may have poor circulation, and any symptoms they have tend to be worse in cold weather. They love warmth and sunshine. Because they are so active and use up so much energy, *Vata* types tend to become dried out. They may get dry skin and hair, but the variability that characterizes them means that some parts of the skin may be dry, while others are oily. Their skin may become wrinkly when they are still comparatively young. Those with high *Vata* tend to suffer from dry bowels and constipation. With their erratic digestions they can suffer from wind, bloating and discomfort and tend to be prone to bowel problems such as irritable bowel syndrome. *Vata* girls tend to have irregular cycles and often miss periods due to stress, overactivity or being underweight; their bleeding tends to be light and may be accompanied by cramping pain.

Vata people are active and restless and find it hard to relax. Their sleep tends to be light and easily disturbed, with many dreams, and they may suffer from nightmares and insomnia. They can easily get overstimulated and drive themselves beyond their energy resources. Their stamina tends to be low and they tire easily, but still push themselves on using their nervous energy until eventually they become exhausted. Vigorous exercise, like running and aerobics, will aggravate their symptoms, even though they may temporarily feel better for it. Gentle exercise such as yoga or t'ai chi is much more suitable, and they need to relax.

When in balance, those with a lot of *Vata* in their constitution are bright, enthusiastic, creative, full of new ideas and initiative, idealistic and visionary. They think fast, talk fast and love being with other people, and enjoy travel and change. They are good at initiating things, but not necessarily at following them through. A clue to their constitution might be gained from observing how many projects they have on the go at any one time, or unfinished books on the bedside table! They are prone to poor memory, lack of concentration, disorganization, fear and anxiety, and can suffer from nervous problems such as disorientation, panic attacks and mood swings.

VATA TRAITS

- A thin frame, erratically proportioned
- Tendency to be underweight or to lose weight when under stress
- Rough, dry skin, which can crack easily; dry hair, bowels, joints, etc.
- Irregular daily routine
- Erratic, fast appetite and digestion
- Love of sweet, sour and salty foods and hot drinks
- Erratic memory, taking things in quickly and forgetting them easily
- Inventive, full of ideas, creative, mentally quick
- Intuitive, highly imaginative, spacey, ungrounded

- Lively, excitable, enthusiastic, changeable, acting on impulse
- Prone to anxiety, fear, insecurity, instability
- Light sleeper, prone to insomnia
- Active, restless, thinking and doing things quickly
- Energetic in bursts, finding it difficult to sustain concentration and activity
- Changeable in mood, with intense feelings
- Easily excited sexually and quickly satiated
- Earns money quickly, spends it quickly
- Feels the cold, often disliking the wind, with symptoms worse in cold weather

- Dreams of running, jumping, flying – often fearful
- Prone to constipation, wind, bloating, headaches, joint pain, muscle tension and spasm, painful periods, infertility, nervous problems, irregular heart rate, dry coughs, insomnia, exhaustion

Pitta

Pitta is a combination of the elements of fire and water. It is the principle of transformation and heat because it is responsible for all the chemical and metabolic conversions in the body that create energy and heat. All *Pitta*'s processes involve digestion or cooking, including the 'cooking' of thoughts into theories in the mind.

Pitta governs our mental analysis, digestion, clarity, perception and understanding. The term comes from the Sanskrit root *tap*, meaning to heat, cook or transform. *Pitta* digests nutrients to provide energy for cellular function; enzymatic and hormonal systems are the main field of *Pitta* activity.

PITTA QUALITIES	
• Oily	• Sharp
• Hot	• Soft
• Light	• Smooth
• Subtle	• Clear
• Flowing	• Malodorous
• Mobile	

In the body *Pitta* governs:
• Appetite, digestion and the metabolism of nutrients
• Thirst
• Body heat and colour
• Lustre of the skin, shine of the hair and light in the eyes.

Mentally and emotionally, *Pitta* governs:
• Mental perception
• Judgment, analysis, discrimination
• Penetrating thought
• Will power, control

- Enthusiasm, joy and courage
- Ambition, competition
- Impatience, irritability, and anger.

The main sites of *Pitta*

The stomach and small intestine are the main sites of *Pitta*, where the digestive acids with their fiery nature create a storehouse of digestive activity. The liver, gall bladder, pancreas and spleen are also the seat of *Pitta*. The blood, containing heat, colour and water, is another province of *Pitta*. The eyes are the sense organ that belongs to the element of fire. Other sites include the skin, brain, sweat and sebaceous glands and hormonal system. *Pitta* is excreted from the body via bile and acid.

Being composed of fire and water, it is the job of *Pitta* to make

Pitta is a combination of fire and water and is responsible for digestion, metabolism and heat.

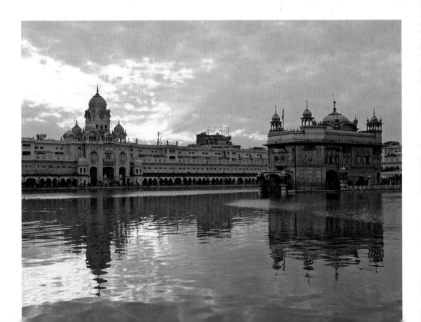

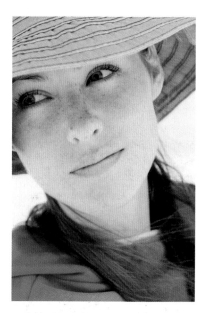

Pitta skin tends to be pale. It burns easily and often has freckles.

Pitta people

Physically, *Pitta*-predominant people tend to be of medium build and weight, with attractive, well-proportioned figures. Their eyes are of medium size, often light in colour and shiny bright; they may be sensitive to sunlight and irritants and may easily become inflamed and watery. Their skin tends to be warm to the touch and pale or pink in appearance; it may be sensitive to heat, sunlight and irritants, and prone to rashes and pimples. The skin burns easily and there are often moles or freckles. *Pitta* types can blush easily or flush with anger. They sweat readily, even in cold weather, and never seem to feel the cold. They are more likely to be intolerant of heat. They may have blond or red hair, which is fine, often straight and oily, and in adulthood turns grey early. Men

two normally antagonistic elements cooperate. All fires in the body, such as digestive acids, are contained in water. If there is more fire than water, the acids will irritate and burn the lining of the stomach or intestine, leading to inflammation, gastritis and ulcers. If there is more water than fire, water drowns out the digestive fire and causes indigestion.

who go bald early are mostly *Pitta* types, as the high levels of testosterone that are associated with baldness are a *Pitta* phenomenon.

Those with high *Pitta* generally have good appetites and love eating. They hate to miss meals and, when hungry, can be irritable and hypoglycaemic, with headaches, dizziness, weakness and shaking. Their digestion is good and their bowels are efficient, but if they get hot, agitated or angry, or eat too many hot, spicy or fried foods, they may suffer from indigestion, heartburn and loose, burning stools. Girls tend to have regular cycles, but may have heavy or long bleeding with bright-red blood, preceded by feeling hot and often irritable premenstrually.

Pitta types are quite methodical and organized. They can be rather obsessive about time and tend to be perfectionists. They often wake up and go to sleep at the same times every day. They sleep well, unless they are worried about something such as work, an interview or public speaking the next day. They are highly competitive and their main fear is of failure. *Pitta* people are naturally intelligent and quite fiery. They can be domineering,

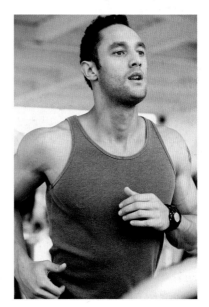

Pitta-*predominant people are highly competitive and love to win.*

critical, self-critical and intolerant. They may suffer from low self-esteem and do not suffer fools gladly.

Hot weather, getting overheated by vigorous exercise, hot, spicy food and red meats can all increase *Pitta*. When *Pitta* is high, it can cause a feeling of increased internal heat, fever and inflammation. Those with an excess of *Pitta* are likely to be irritable, angry, overly critical and achievement-oriented, and there is a tendency to be a workaholic. Various acids or bile accumulate in the tissues, causing fermentation, infection and skin disorders like herpes, eczema and acne. Bleeding (as in nosebleeds or heavy periods) and excessive discharges of sweat or urine often occur. High *Pitta* causes yellow coloration of the stool, urine, eyes and skin, strong-smelling secretions of sweat and urine, excessive hunger and thirst, burning sensations in the body and difficulty in sleeping.

PITTA TRAITS

- **Medium build and weight, strong and well built**
- **Regular features, well-proportioned body**
- **Smooth, oily skin, fair or reddish, often with moles and freckles, which burns easily; hot to the touch**
- **Bright, penetrating eyes, which are sensitive to smoke and sunlight**
- **Good, strong appetite, fast metabolism**
- **Good digestion, with a tendency to low blood sugar, which can cause irritability or headaches**
- **Fine shiny hair, which falls out easily and goes grey early; men are prone to baldness**
- **Profuse perspiration, with smelly secretions**
- **Cravings for sweet, salty, pungent and sour foods and cold drinks**

- Highly intelligent, sharp mind, good memory and concentration
- Tends to be irritable, angry, impatient, intolerant and judgmental
- Perfectionist, organized and efficient
- Decisive, assertive, ambitious, competitive and entrepreneurial
- Good at public speaking
- Likes to be in control, has leadership qualities, can be authoritarian
- Anxious about not getting things right, not being in control, fearful of failure
- Passionate, romantic, intense, can be obsessive
- Sexually energetic, can be dominating
- May suffer from lack of self-esteem, depression and jealousy
- Dreams of fire, war, aggression, competition
- Likes to earn and spend money, loves to wear or surround themselves with beautiful things
- Dislikes intense heat, with symptoms often worse in hot weather or if overheated
- Goes to bed late, tends to work into the night; sleep is of medium duration
- Prone to inflammatory problems, heat and burning symptoms, skin rashes, infections and fevers, heartburn and indigestion, peptic ulcers, loose bowels, sore, irritated eyes, visual problems, anaemia, liver or gall-bladder problems

Kapha

Kapha **is a combination of earth and water, the principle of potential energy, of growth and protection. Kapha is responsible for the body's nourishment and makes up the bulk of our structure – the bones, muscles, tissues, cells and body fluids.**

In the body *Kapha* governs:
• Strength and stability
• The water balance of the body
• Lubrication of the mucous membranes and the joints (synovial membranes)
• Protecting and cushioning the whole body
• Supporting and holding the structures of the body together.

On a psychological level *Kapha* provides:
• Emotional support in life
• Calmness and endurance
• Patience and forgiveness
• The ability to feel love, compassion and devotion
• A sense of well-being
• Loyalty and affection.

KAPHA QUALITIES

• Wet	• Static
• Cold	• Dull
• Gross	• Soft
• Dense	• Cloudy
• Smooth	• Heavy

The main sites of *Kapha*

The primary site of *Kapha* is the stomach. The chest or lungs produce phlegm, as do the throat, head, sinuses and nasal passages, which are all also *Kapha* sites. The mouth and tongue produce saliva, another *Kapha* fluid. The

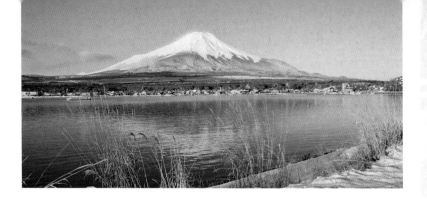

tongue is the organ of taste, the sense that belongs to the water element. Fat tissue, brain tissue, the joints, the lymph, the pancreas and the pleural and pericardial cavities are also the province of *Kapha*. These are the areas where *Kapha* disorders will generally manifest. *Kapha* is excreted from the body via mucus.

Kapha keeps the body's earth suspended in its water. It enables water and earth, which would not otherwise interact with one another, to combine properly and remain in balance. The physical body is composed mainly of water and is contained within the boundaries of the skin and other tissue linings (earth). Earth alone

Kapha is a combination of the elements of water and earth and makes up the bulk of our physical structure.

is immobile and, as such, can block organic functions and predispose one to disease; only in solution in water does it function in the body.

If the body becomes too solid, with an excess of earth element, problems such as gall stones and kidney stones develop. These stones are concentrations of earth in which the water has dried out too much to permit free flow to continue. If there is too much water and not enough earth in the system, disturbances like oedema can develop.

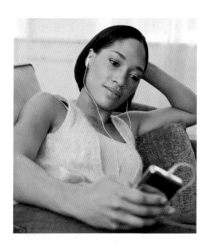

Kapha types like nothing better than sitting around and relaxing.

Kapha people

Kapha-predominant people tend to be grounded, emotionally and physically strong, and resilient. They are placid, kind and thoughtful. They tend to be sweet-natured, loyal and affectionate and will often avoid confrontation. They don't like change or the unpredictable aspects of life, and will do anything to maintain the status quo. They may have a tendency to be lazy – 'couch potatoes' who like nothing better than sitting around, relaxing and doing very little. Exerting themselves often does not come naturally, although vigorous exercise can make them feel very good and healthy.

Physically, *Kapha*-predominant people have the biggest and strongest builds of all three types, and *Kapha* women tend to be the most fertile. They tend to have large bones, broad shoulders and big muscles and to put on weight easily. Their hair is thick and lustrous, their eyes calm, large and moist, their nails wide and strong, their lips full and their teeth strong and even. Their appetite is stable, though they are often not hungry first thing in the morning, when they tend to feel sleepy. They love food and have a tendency to comfort eat. Their digestion is slow and sluggish, as is their metabolism. They sleep heavily and love to lie in. Their skin is usually cool and rather clammy to the touch, and they don't tend to mind extremes of weather, but their symptoms (such as colds and mucous congestion) are often worse in cold, damp, winter weather.

Kapha tends to accumulate during cold, damp weather in winter and early spring. It is also increased by a sedentary life, lack of exercise and eating too many sweet foods and carbohydrates. *Kapha* promotes stasis, which can lead to inertia. Those with excess *Kapha* may feel slow, heavy, lethargic and inactive, and have a tendency to accumulate more earth and water – that is, to put on weight and retain

Kapha people tend to have thick hair and full lips; they love food and have a tendency to comfort eat.

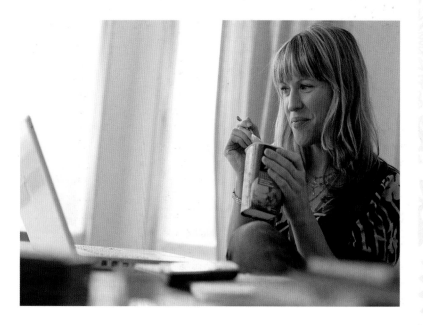

water. Emotionally they may feel complacent, greedy, materialistic, acquisitive, attached, possessive, and mentally passive, slow and dull. There may be a tendency to be stubborn, obstinate and narrow-minded and to block out any unpleasant or disturbing thoughts or emotions that might upset their equilibrium. They would be reluctant to delve into their emotional life in counselling or psychotherapy. They can feel low and unmotivated, especially in winter, and can suffer from depression and seasonal affective disorder (SAD), sometimes spending hours doing very little.

Excess *Kapha* can predispose one to stagnation in the tissues, lymphatic congestion, cellulite, mucous congestion, breathing problems, pallor, feeling cold, sleepiness and low thyroid function. Too much *Kapha* is associated with low digestive fire, causing heaviness in the stomach, nausea after eating and sluggish bowels.

KAPHA TRAITS

- Large frame, heavy bones, big muscles
- Thick, lustrous, oily skin and hair
- Large, clear eyes, full lips, large, strong teeth
- Strong physique and immunity, good resistance to disease
- Energy is steady and enduring – the strongest of all the constitutions
- Tendency to oversleep, to be lazy and inactive
- Slow digestion and metabolism
- Craving for sweet, sour and salty foods
- Prone to being overweight, feeling heavy
- Slow-moving and graceful
- Calm, easy-going, slow-paced, mild and gentle
- Methodical, slow and deliberate

- Resistant to change, stubborn, slow to react, blocking out difficult emotions; may be in denial
- Loyal and dependable, non-judgmental, and disliking change
- Calm, grounded, affectionate, forgiving and compassionate, striving to maintain stability inside and around them
- Voluptuous, but slow to arouse sexually and then strong and enduring
- Slow to learn and slow to forget
- Tends to be acquisitive, greedy, possessive and clingy
- Good at earning money and saving
- Feels worse in cold, damp weather
- Sleeps long and deeply; hard to wake in the morning
- Dreams of water, nature, birds and gentle romantic images
- Prone to colds, catarrhal congestion, asthma, lethargy, low motivation and depression, lymphatic congestion, being overweight, allergies, high cholesterol and diabetes

Relationships and the *doshas*

Kapha serves as a support and a vehicle for the other two *doshas*, Vata and Pitta. It acts as a conserving and restraining force on them and their active and consuming effect on body and mind, which may otherwise disperse and dissipate vital energy.

The subtle energy of *Kapha* is called *Ojas*, which is the prime energy reserve in the body responsible for our strength, vitality, immunity and fertility. When *Kapha* is low, due to high *Vata* or *Pitta* (through stress, poor diet, illness and so on), our immunity as well as the emotional and mental well-being that *Kapha* engenders will be compromised.

Vata and Kapha are almost opposite each other in quality:
- **Kapha** represents all potential states of energy in the body and permits energy to be stored
- **Vata** represents all kinetic states of energy in the body and causes stored energy to be released
- **Pitta** balances between change

Kapha *governs the first stage of life, from birth to the age of 16.*

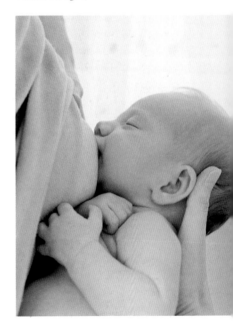

and stasis, overstimulation and inertia.

Vata and *Kapha* congregate near each other in the body for practical reasons. The heart and lungs are continuously in motion and so require continuous lubrication. Too much motion uses up the lubricant, while too much lubricant gums up the works. In the joints the synovial fluid provides lubrication and protection. The brain and spinal cord, whose movement manifests as nerve impulses, swim in cerebrospinal fluid. Mucus protects the lining of the gut, enabling the food to pass through it freely.

The cycle of human existence

Kapha dosha is responsible for the growth of children to physical maturity, from birth to the age of 16; *Pitta dosha* is responsible for the maintenance of the body in its maturity, aged 16–45; and *Vata dosha* is responsible for the decline of the body, from the age of 45 to death. These cycles can be extended as we achieve greater longevity, so that the *Pitta* cycle could continue in some people until the age of 50 or 55.

To be healthy, the balance of the *doshas* that we have at birth needs to be maintained. If the balance is disturbed by diet, weather, season, lifestyle or state of mind, illness eventually results and may be felt as physical discomfort and pain or as mental and emotional suffering. The current state of imbalance causing such symptoms to manifest is known as our *Vikruti*.

When it comes to treatment, sensitive *Vata* types generally need smaller doses of medicine and benefit from warming, nourishing and calming herbs. More robust *Pitta* types can be given medium doses and more cooling and detoxifying herbs; slow-reacting *Kapha* types may require higher doses of warming, energizing and decongestant herbs over a longer period of time.

The five subtypes of the *doshas*

There are five types of each *dosha*, which reside in different places in the body and are responsible for different vital functions. Through them you can understand and treat the *doshas* more specifically.

The five types of *Vata*

The five forms of *Vata* are of prime importance, as *Prana* (the first type of *Vata*) is the life force – the motivating energy that underlies all activities. The Sanskrit names are formed by adding different prefixes to the root *an*, which means 'to breathe or energize'. The forms of *Vata* are also called *Vayu*, another word meaning 'wind'.

Prana Vata

Prana Vata or *Vayu* – the cosmic life energy and our life force – is the primary wind or energy in the body, which directs all the other types of *Vata*. The prefix *Pra* means 'inward' or 'toward'. It is located in the head, particularly in the brain,

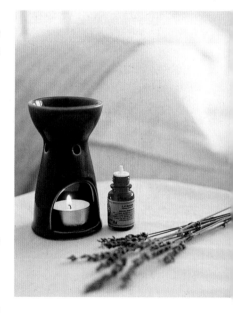

Therapeutic methods such as aromatherapy and Pranayama *can be used to strengthen* Prana *when it is impaired.*

and moves inward and downward to the chest and throat, governing inhalation and swallowing. *Prana Vata* governs consciousness, the mind, heart and the senses, gives us inspiration in life and connects us with our inner self and pure consciousness.

Prana brings air and food into the body and enables us to take in impressions, feelings and information. It governs our ability to be receptive to external and internal forms of nourishment, including our inner connection to the cosmic life force. When *Prana* is sufficient it is said that we are immune to all disease. When it is impaired we become prone to ill health, which can be treated by therapeutic methods such as *Pranayama* (breathing exercises) and aromatherapy, which strengthen it.

Udana Vata

Udana Vata or *Vayu* is 'upward- or outward-moving air' (*ud* means 'upward'). It resides in the chest and is centred in the throat, and governs exhalation and speech, and various forms of exertion that occur through the outgoing breath, including singing. Its action is to move energy from the inside to the outside. *Udana Vata* is said to cause our minds and spirits to ascend. It is responsible for enthusiasm, good memory, strength, motivation and effort, and governs our aspirations and self-expression. It promotes higher values and, when fully developed, gives us the power to transcend the outer world. When impaired, *Udana Vata* can cause speech problems, coughing, sneezing, yawning, belching and vomiting. The practice of yoga promotes the development of *Udana Vata*.

Samana Vata

Samana Vata or *Vayu* means 'equalizing air'. *Sama* means 'balancing' or 'equalizing' (as in our word 'same'). Its function is to balance the inner and outer, upper and lower parts of the body and their energies in the process of digestion. Our minds and emotions need to be in balance to absorb nutrients on all levels. It has some ascending action.

Located in the stomach and small intestine, *Samana Vata* is the nervous force behind digestion, governing the absorption of energy via the digestive system and the assimilation of nutrients. When its function is impaired it causes lack of appetite or nervous indigestion.

Vyana Vata

Vyana Vata or *Vayu* means 'diffusive air' or 'pervasive air'. *Vi* means 'to separate'. *Vyana Vata* is located in the heart and circulated throughout the body. It has a mainly outward action, which enables us to express ourselves in action and to release energy. It governs the circulatory system, the blood supply through the body

and specifically to the muscles, enabling the use of energy through muscular exertion. Its action is mainly in the limbs, the prime site of movement in the body.

Disturbance of *Vyana Vata* can cause poor coordination and difficulty moving, particularly walking. Too much *Vyana Vata* can overly diffuse or disperse our energy. It is the opposite of *Prana*, which is inward-moving.

Apana Vata

Apana Vata or *Vayu* means 'downward-moving air'. *Apa* means 'moving away', as *Apana Vata* governs the elimination of waste energy. It is located in the lower abdomen and colon, and is responsible for all downward-moving impulses of elimination, including defecation, urination, menstruation, parturition and sex. When impaired it affects these functions and causes symptoms such as constipation, diarrhoea and painful periods. It also governs the absorption of water in

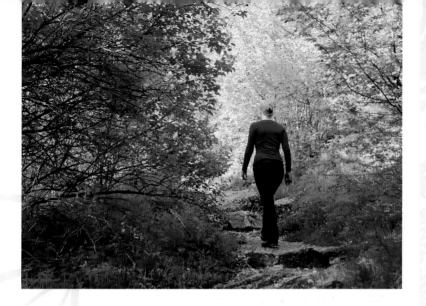

Vyana Vata supplies blood to the muscles, enabling the use of energy through muscular exertion.

the large intestine, and enables us to take in full nourishment from the digestion of food, the final stage of which occurs in the large intestine.

Apana Vata supports and controls all other forms of *Vata*, and an imbalance forms the basis of most *Vata* disorders. So treatment of *Apana Vata* is the first consideration in the treatment of *Vata*, and enables the other *Vatas* to return to normal functioning. *Vata* disorders are the fundamental basis of most diseases and always accompany those of *Pitta* and *Kapha*. For this reason it is always important to consider *Apana* in the treatment of any disease. Keeping all five *Vatas* in balance and properly functioning is the vital key to maintaining health. *Apana* is like the plug on the body's energy, which can be opened to let waste energy out, but if left open will drain *Prana* from the body.

The five types of *Pitta*

These are sometimes referred to as *Agnis* (fires) as they all serve to provide or promote fire, digestion, heat and transformation on various levels of body and mind.

Sadhaka Pitta

Sadhaka means 'the fire that tells truth from reality', from the root *sadh*, meaning 'to accomplish' or 'to realize'. It is the fire in the brain and heart and functions through the nervous system and senses, and is responsible for intelligence and the attainment of intellectual as well as spiritual goals. On a material level these goals might be pleasure, wealth and prestige.

Sadhaka Pitta governs mental energy, the digestion of impressions, ideas or beliefs and

Disturbance of Sadhaka Pitta *can cause confusion, over-analysing, low self-esteem and depression.*

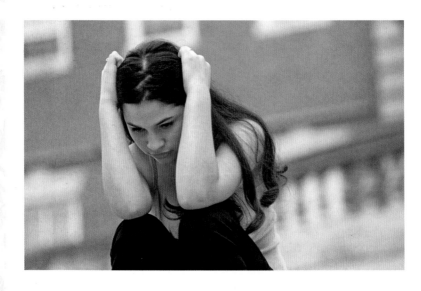

our power of discrimination. It has an inward movement, governing the release of energy from our impressions and life experiences to empower the mind. It directs our intelligence within. When it is impaired we suffer from lack of clarity, confusion, delusion, insomnia, anger, intolerance, depression (which can be severe) and low self-esteem.

Alochaka Pitta

This governs visual perception. It is located in the eyes and is responsible for the reception of light from the world around us, the digestion of impressions and vision. Centred in the pupil, it allows us to see and connects our eyes to our emotions. It has an upward movement stimulating us to seek light, clarity and understanding to feed the mind and soul. Clearness in the eyes is a sign of good digestion and liver function, mental clarity and higher intelligence. When *Alochaka Pitta* is disturbed we may suffer from eye problems such

as conjunctivitis and visual problems such as photophobia.

Pachaka Pitta

Located in the small intestine, *Pachaka Pitta* governs the enzymes that enable digestion to take place. It is also responsible for the regulation of temperature and the maintenance of good circulation. When it is too high it can cause indigestion, hyperacidity and ulcers, and when it is too low it can cause poor absorption and lack of body heat.

Pachaka Pitta is the main form of *Pitta* and the support for all other *Pittas*. It is the first consideration when treating *Pitta*, as our primary source of heat is the digestive fire, *Agni*. Through its power of discrimination it can separate the nutrient from the non-nutrient part of food and is responsible for the absorption of nutrients, as well as for local immunity in the gastrointestinal tract, destroying pathogens that enter the body with food.

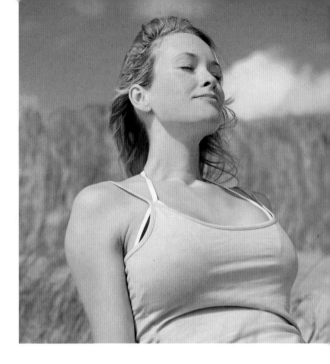

Brajaka Pitta *is responsible for the complexion and colour of our skin.*

Brajaka Pitta

Brajaka Pitta means 'the fire that governs lustre or complexion', and is located in the skin. It is responsible for the temperature, complexion and colour of our skin. When aggravated, it causes rashes and discoloration. *Brajaka Pitta* governs the absorption of warmth, heat and sunlight through the skin and has an outward-moving action, through which heat can be diffused by means of the circulation.

Ranjaka Pitta

Ranjaka Pitta means 'the fire that imparts colour'. It is located in the liver, spleen, stomach and small intestine, colouring the blood, bile and stool, as well as other waste materials. Its main site is the blood, where it gives warmth and colour. It has downward-moving energy.

The five types of *Kapha*

These protect our organs and tissues from wear and tear caused by the drying effect of *Vata* and the heat of *Pitta*. They help to maintain cohesion and strength.

Tarpaka Kapha

Located in the brain and heart in the form of cerebrospinal fluid, *Tarpaka Kapha* affords protection, strength, nourishment and lubrication to the nerves. It cushions them from the effects of stress, promoting emotional calm and stability, as well as happiness and good memory. A deficiency of *Tarpaka Kapha* can cause discontent, malaise, nervousness and insomnia. It has an inward movement, enabling us to feel the inner joy of being ourselves. Meditation promotes its secretion.

Bodhaka Kapha

This means 'the form of water that gives perception'. It is located in the mouth and tongue as the saliva that enables us to taste our food, as part of the first stage of digestion. It also protects the mouth from irritation by harsh, pungent foods and drinks. A deranged sense of taste often precedes *Kapha* disorders. It has upward-moving action and governs the sense of taste in our life and our refinement of taste as we evolve.

Meditation promotes the secretion of Tarpaka Kapha, which provides strength and nourishment to the nervous system.

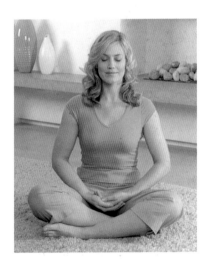

Kledaka Kapha

This means 'the water that moistens'. It is located in the stomach as the alkaline secretions of the mucous membranes, and is responsible for the moistening of food and for the first stage of digestion. It also protects the delicate mucous membranes. Impairment of *Kledaka Kapha* manifests as the irregular secretion of stomach fluids and excess phlegm.

Sleshaka Kapha

This means 'water that gives lubrication', from the root *slish*, meaning 'to be moist or sticky'. It is located in the joints as synovial fluid, where it is responsible for holding them together and easing movement by preventing friction. Impairment of *Sleshaka Kapha* causes drying out of the synovial fluid, leading to dry, cracking joints and predisposing to arthritis. It has an outward action, giving us strength and stability for physical movement.

Avalambaka Kapha

This means 'the water that gives support'. It is located in the heart and lungs, where it provides lubrication. *Avalambaka Kapha* corresponds to basic plasma, *Rasa*, which is distributed by lung and heart action, from which all *Kapha* is produced. It is the main form of *Kapha* and supports the actions of the other *Kaphas*, so it is the most important aspect of *Kapha* in the treatment of disease.

Avalambaka Kapha has a downward action, and gives support. If it is excessive it can cause us to feel heavy, overweight and prone to pulmonary disorders. Derangement of *Avalambaka Kapha* lies behind most accumulations of phlegm in the body. Clearing the chest of phlegm is the basis for removing *Kapha* from the entire body, including water retention.

The five types of Kapha *help maintain cohesion and strength.*

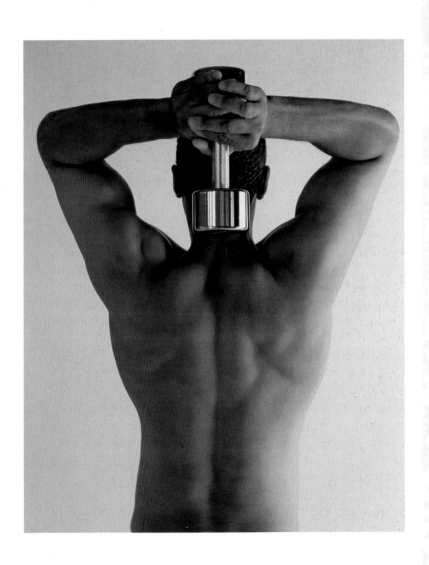

The seven tissues

According to Ayurveda, the human body is composed of seven tissue layers or *dhatus* (from the root *dha*, meaning 'to support'). While the balance of the *doshas* can predispose to ill health, the *dhatus* can become the sites of disease, in which case they are called *dushya*, meaning 'that which can be spoiled'. For health and strength, the seven *dhatus* need to be functioning optimally.

The *dhatus* are formed from digested nutrients, and the waste products of their metabolism are eliminated though faeces and urine. *Rasa* is the first *dhatu* and consists of the basic plasma of the body from which all other tissues are produced. Each tissue is produced by digestion out of the other, so that each one becomes food for the next; this means there is only one tissue in the body that undergoes seven levels of transformation, so problems in any one tissue can easily affect all the rest. From the gross to the most subtle, the seven *dhatus* are:

- *Rasa* (plasma) – composed primarily of water
- *Rakta* (blood, specifically haemoglobin) – composed of fire and water
- *Mamsa* (muscle, skeletal and visceral) – composed primarily of earth and secondarily of water and fire
- *Medas* (fat or adipose tissue) – composed mainly of water
- *Asthi* (bone) – composed of earth and air
- *Majja* (marrow and nerve tissue) – composed of water and earth
- *Shukra* (reproductive tissue) – the essence derived from all tissues.

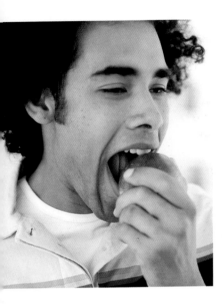

The seven dhatus *are formed from digested nutrients.*

tissue is formed from the one that precedes it, so it takes 35 days to make *Shukra* (reproductive tissue).

Rasa (plasma)

Rasa means both 'essence/sap' and 'to circulate'. It provides nutrition for the five elements in the body and nourishment to all the tissues. *Rasa* is responsible for tissue hydration and for maintaining electrolyte balance. Psychologically, when *Rasa* is sufficient we feel happy and content, with enthusiasm, vitality and compassion for others. Our complexion is good, and our skin and hair are soft and shiny. *Rasa* circulates around the whole body, but the main sites are the heart, blood vessels, lymphatic system, skin and mucous membranes. *Rasa* (plasma) and *Kapha* are closely related, as *Kapha* is contained in *Rasa* (plasma).

As it is the basic substance of the body, *Kapha* is responsible for all *dhatus* generally, and specifically for five: *Rasa* (plasma); *Mamsa* (muscle); *Medas* (fat); *Majja* (marrow); and *Shukra* (reproductive tissue). *Pitta* governs *Rakta* (blood) and *Vata* governs *Asthi* (bone).

Rasa (plasma) is formed daily from our food, and from it the next tissue *Rakta* (blood) is formed. This process takes five days. Each

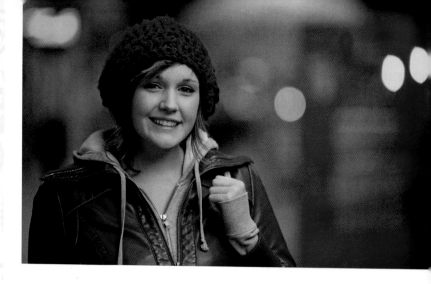

When Rakta *is sufficient our skin is warm and radiant.*

Excess *Rasa* from, for instance, overeating creates an increase of *Kapha* and an accumulation of saliva and mucus, which can block channels (*srotas*) and cause loss of appetite and nausea. Deficiency of *Rasa* causes dry skin and lips, dehydration, tiredness after slight exertion, intolerance of noise, tremors, palpitations, aches and pain due to poor nourishment of all the subsequent *dhatus*.

Rakta (blood tissue)

This is composed of fire and water. It is both a fluid and a conveyor of heat because it contains haemoglobin, which carries oxygen for cell respiration. *Rakta* means 'what is coloured' or 'what is red'. It gives us colour both literally and figuratively. When *Rakta* is sufficient our life energy is good, and we have passion for life, faith and love. The skin is warm and radiant, the lips and tongue are a healthy pink and the conjunctiva of the eyes is clear.

Rakta corresponds to *Pitta*, as *Pitta* is carried in the blood.

Excess *Rakta* causes skin problems, boils and abscesses, enlargement of the liver and spleen, hypertension, jaundice, digestive problems, burning sensations, and redness or bleeding in the skin, eyes and urine. Deficiency of *Rakta* causes pallor, low blood pressure, a desire for sour and cold food, dry and dull hair and skin, and capillary fragility.

Mamsa (muscle tissue)

This is composed primarily of earth, along with secondary water and fire. It is heavy and makes up much of the bulk of the body. *Mamsa* comes from the root *man*, meaning 'to hold firm', as the muscles serve to hold the basic body frame together and give it strength. When *Mamsa* is deficient we lack the strength and cohesion that enable us to work hard and exercise. When *Mamsa* is sufficient it gives us courage, confidence and endurance, with the ability to be open, compassionate, forgiving and happy.

Excess *Mamsa* creates swelling or tumours in the muscles, swollen glands, obesity, liver enlargement, irritability and aggression. In women it could lead to the development of fibroids, a tendency to miscarriage and low sexual energy. Deficiency of *Mamsa* leads to weakness, poor muscle tone and wasting, particularly around the hips, abdomen and the back of the neck, lack of coordination, fear, insecurity and anxiety.

Medas (fat tissue)

This is mainly composed of water. Its function is lubrication and protection throughout the body. It helps lubricate the throat to enable a good singing voice; it also oils the skin, the hair and the eyes. *Medas* promotes a feeling of ease, comfort, joy and a sense of well-being and protection. Those who don't feel loved or protected may surround themselves with a layer of fat and become obese.

Excess *Medas* leads to lethargy, heaviness, poor mobility, asthma and low sexual energy, as well as thirst, hypertension, diabetes, poor longevity and sagging of the thighs, breasts and belly. Emotionally it is related to being closed-minded, attached and possessive. Deficiency of *Medas* causes cracking joints, loss of weight, dry and brittle hair, nails, teeth and bones and fatigue, as well as feelings of fear, anger and anxiety.

Asthi (bone tissue)

This is composed of earth, which is the solid part of bone, and air, its porosity. The word *Asthi* comes from the root *stha*, meaning 'to stand or endure', as its function is to support the body and give it a strong foundation. When *Asthi* is sufficient it promotes fortitude, stamina, stability, confidence and certainty. It gives strong bones and flexible movement of the joints, as well as strong white teeth. *Asthi* is

related to *Vata*, as *Vata* is contained in the bone tissue. Excess *Asthi* creates extra bone tissue, spurs, extra teeth, an over-large frame, joint pain, fear, anxiety and poor stamina. Deficiency of *Asthi* creates tiredness, joint pain or

Regular weight-bearing exercise such as yoga helps to promote and preserve good Asthi dhatu.

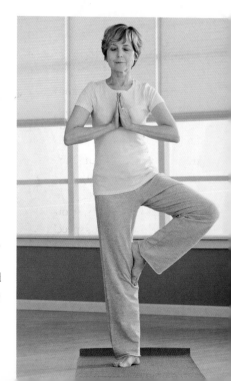

weakness, hair loss, poor formation of bones, nails and teeth, and osteoporosis.

Majja (marrow and nerve tissue)

This is composed of a subtle form of water and some earth. *Majja* comes from the root *maj*, meaning 'to sink', as the bone marrow and nerve tissue are found inside the spinal cord and bones. Its function is to fill the empty spaces in the body, including the nerve channels, bones and brain cavity. It also makes up synovial fluid and aids the lubrication of the eyes, stool and skin, as well as the production of red blood cells. On a psychological level, *Majja* promotes adaptability, receptivity, affection and compassion. Healthy *Majja* is indicated by clear eyes, strong joints, good powers of speech and tolerance of pain. The mind is sharp and clear and the memory is good.

Excess *Majja* creates heaviness of the eyes, limbs and joints, deep non-healing sores, and infections in the eyes. A deficiency creates weak, porous bones, pain in the joints, dizziness, spots before the eyes, darkness around the eyes, sexual debility, feeling ungrounded, and poor concentration and memory.

Shukra (reproductive tissue)

This is the essential tissue form of water that has the power to create new life. *Shukra* means 'seed' and 'luminous' and is also the Sanskrit name for the planet Venus. It includes the ovum, sperm and reproductive fluids. When it is healthy, *Shukra* provides strength, energy and vitality for the entire body. It offers strong immunity, well-formed secondary sex characteristics, and a loving and compassionate nature. It gives light to the eyes and inspiration to the soul and is essential to fertility.

Excess *Shukra* creates excessive sexual desire, often leading to

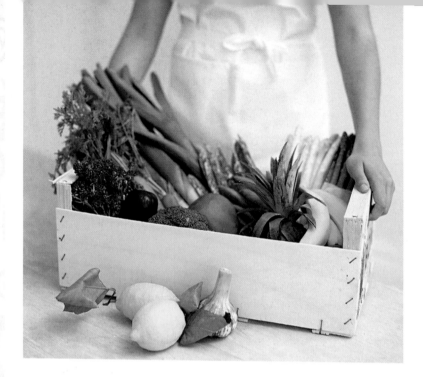

frustration, excess semen, stones in the semen and enlargement of the prostate. Deficiency creates a lack of sexual energy and arousal, infertility, insecurity, impotence, frigidity and anxiety.

The dhatus *are formed from digested food and ideally this should contain all the nutrients necessary for each* dhatu.

Ojas

This is the eighth tissue, a super-fine essence of all *dhatus*. It is the subtle essence of all *Kapha* or water in the body, particularly the essence of the reproductive fluid. It is the ultimate product of nutrition and digestion, as well as the prime energy reserve for the whole body. It gives us immunity, strength, resilience, fertility and longevity.

Formation of the *dhatus*

The *dhatus* are formed from digested food, which is known as the nutrient chyle or *Ahararasa*, and ideally this should contain all the necessary nutrients for each *dhatu*. The *Ahararasa* is carried to the liver, where it is further metabolized and broken down into the five basic elements (ether, air, fire, water and earth) that provide the building blocks for the seven *dhatus*.

Each *dhatu* has its own individual *Agni*, or digestive fire, which is known as a tissue fire or *dhatu-Agni*. This ensures that the appropriate nutrients are metabolized from the *Ahararasa* for each *dhatu*.

The nutrient chyle or *Ahararasa* provides nourishment for each *dhatu*. Each *dhatu* is made up of two parts, one stable and the other in formation of the next *dhatu*.

The unstable portion of one *dhatu* is transformed by the *dhatu-Agni* of the succeeding *dhatu* and becomes the stable form of the subsequent *dhatu*. To illustrate this, from the *Ahararasa* is formed the first *dhatu*, *Rasa*. Half of it remains in a stable form and the other half, as the unstable portion, is acted on by *Rakta-dhatu-Agni* and is transformed into *Rakta dhatu*.

A secondary tissue called an *upadhatu* is created. Blood vessels and tendons are the *upadhatu* of *Rakta dhatu*.

A waste portion known as a *kittapaka* is produced; *Pitta* is the waste product of *Rakta dhatu* formation.

Then half of the *dhatu* – in this case *Rakta dhatu* – remains in its stable form, and from the unstable portion the next *dhatu* is formed, in this case *Mamsa dhatu*.

The adequate formation of a *dhatu* depends on the previous tissue being properly formed, and the tissue *Agni* must function normally. If the *dhatu Agni* is too low, an excess of the tissue will be produced and its quality will be poor. If the tissue *Agni* is too high, then a deficiency of the *dhatu* will be produced as it is burned up.

In this process of tissue formation, secondary tissues known as *upadhatus* are produced – like menstrual fluid from plasma. Waste materials are also produced, like *Kapha* from *Rasa*/plasma.

The waste product (mala) of Majja dhatu *is tears and eye secretions.*

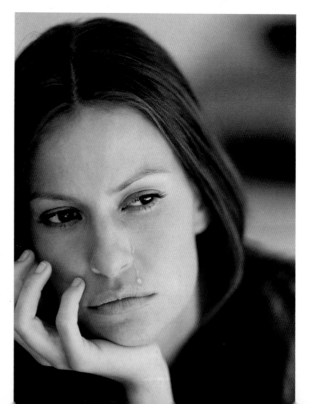

UPADHATUS/SECONDARY TISSUES

- **Plasma** – breast milk and menstrual flow
- **Blood** – blood vessels and tendons
- **Muscles** – ligaments and skin
- **Fat** – the omentum (the layer of fat covering the abdomen)
- **Bone** – the teeth
- **Marrow** – the sclerotic fluid in the eyes
- **Reproductive tissue** – *Ojas*

MALAS/WASTE PRODUCTS OF TISSUE METABOLISM

- **Plasma** – *Kapha* (phlegm)
- **Blood** – *Pitta* (bile)
- **Muscles** – waste material in the outer cavities like the ear (e.g. ear wax)
- **Fat** – sweat
- **Bone** – nails and hair
- **Marrow** – tears and eye secretions
- **Reproductive tissue** – smegma (waste material secreted by the genitals)

Dhatu development

To produce healthy tissues and thereby keep ourselves functioning optimally it is vital that the food we eat is of top quality. Next, our digestive fire needs to be able to digest the ingested food into the nutrient chyle and the *dhatu-Agni* need to be firing well. The strength of the tissue digestive fire (*dhatu-Agni*) determines the quality and quantity of tissue produced. Over-high tissue fire causes deficient formation of the tissue, due to hypermetabolism; and low *Agni* causes the formation of an excess of poor-quality tissue. When too little of a *dhatu* is formed, or it is of a poor quality, it is unable to nourish the next one, which is subsequently depleted also, and so on down the line.

Kapha and *Pitta* in normal amounts not only produce *Rasa* and *Rakta*, but also their excess is excreted as waste materials. So, when these two *dhatus* are excessive, *Kapha* and *Pitta* will be overproduced too. Most *Kapha* diseases involve *Rasa*, and *Pitta* diseases involve *Rakta*. *Vata* is closely related to *Asthi* (bone) and contained within it. Many *Vata* diseases involve the bones, such as arthritis and osteoporosis. Most deficient states of the *dhatus* present as *Vata* symptoms.

Kapha types tend to have well-developed *dhatus*, but tend toward excess. Their blood and bone (the *Pitta* and *Vata dhatus*) tend to be deficient. Overdevelopment of *Rasa* and production of excess phlegm may block development of the next tissue, *Rakta*. Overdevelopment of muscle tends to cause underdevelopment of the next tissues, the fat and reproductive tissues, while overdevelopment of *Medas* blocks the development of bone, marrow and reproductive tissue. Under-production of a tissue will also block the formation of subsequent tissues. It will fail to nourish more subtle *dhatus* and to support the other more gross ones.

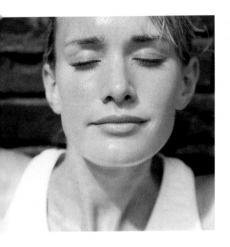

Sweating helps cool the body and clear excess fat and toxins from it.

Malas

There are three primary waste materials (*malas*):

- Faeces (*Purisha*)
- Urine (*Mutra*)
- Sweat (*Sveda*).

Not only do the *malas* ensure elimination of waste products from the body, but they also fulfil other functions. Faeces maintain the tone and temperature of the colon and discharge excess earth and air from the body. Urine carries acids from the blood (*Pitta*), as does sweat, and aids blood purification. Sweat aids cooling of the body and moistens the skin and surface hair; it also clears excess fat from the body. All three *malas* aid the elimination of excess heat from the body.

Malas can themselves be damaged by excess *doshas* and *dhatus*, which inhibit their eliminative functions. If *malas* are not released, they accumulate and affect the surrounding tissues. Excess faeces cause abdominal pain, constipation, headache and toxicity. Excess urine causes bladder pain, irritable bladder and water retention. Excess sweat causes body odour and skin disease. Excess *Pitta* is involved with skin diseases like urticaria, eczema and boils. Often excess sweating, particularly in *Vata* people, can cause dehydration and fatigue.

The 20 attributes

From the three *gunas* come the 20 main attributes – which are ten pairs of opposites, being the positive and negative aspects of all forces and material objects in the universe.

The 10 pairs of opposites are:
- cold/hot (*shita/ushna*)
- static/mobile (*sthira/chala*)
- wet/dry (*snigda/ruksha*)
- dull/sharp (*manda/tikshna*)
- heavy/light (*guru/laghu*)
- soft/hard (*mridu/kathina*)
- gross/subtle (*sthula/sukshma*)
- smooth/rough (*slakshna/khara*)
- dense/flowing (*sandra/drava*)
- cloudy/clear (*picchila/vishada*)

In nature and the body, cold, wet, heavy, gross and dense qualities go together, as do hot, dry, light, subtle and flowing qualities. The former tend to descend and contract and serve to create the body, as we see in *Kapha*. The latter ascend and expand and create energy, vitality and mental perception.

Foods and herbs all have these qualities and can be used to correct imbalances of these qualities. Generally speaking, like increases like, so a food or herb with cold, wet, heavy qualities will increase those qualities in *Kapha* types. Therapeutically it is opposites that are employed, so that cinnamon (with its hot, dry, mobile and clear qualities) will help disperse the cold, heavy, solid, static and dull qualities of winter that may otherwise increase *Kapha* symptoms.

The box opposite shows the qualities of the *doshas* and elements and the attributes of the *gunas*. The qualities of *Tamas* resemble those of the earth element; the qualities of *Rajas* resemble those of fire; those of *Sattva* are like ether.

THE *DOSHAS*, ELEMENTS AND *GUNAS*

Qualities of the *doshas*

- *Vata*: cold, light, dry, subtle, mobile, sharp, hard, rough, clear
- *Pitta*: hot, a little wet, light, subtle, flowing, mobile, sharp, soft, smooth, clear
- *Kapha*: cold, wet, heavy, gross, dense, static, dull, soft, smooth, cloudy

Qualities of the elements

- **Ether**: cold, dry, light, subtle, mobile, sharp, soft, smooth, clear
- **Air**: cold, dry, light, subtle, mobile, sharp, rough, hard, clear
- **Fire**: hot, dry, light, subtle, mobile, sharp, rough, hard, clear
- **Water**: cold, wet, heavy, gross, liquid, static, dull, soft, smooth, cloudy
- **Earth**: cold, dry, heavy, gross, solid, static, dull, hard, rough, cloudy

Attributes of the *gunas*

- *Sattva*: neither hot nor cold, neither wet nor dry, light, subtle, mobile, sharp, soft, smooth, clear
- *Rajas*: hot, a little wet, slightly heavy, gross, mobile, sharp, hard, rough, cloudy
- *Tamas*: cold, wet, heavy, gross, solid, static, dull, hard, rough, cloudy

Srotas: the channels of circulation

According to Ayurveda, the body contains innumerable channels called *srotas*, through which the basic tissue elements, *doshas* and *malas* circulate. They are present throughout the visible and invisible body of cells, molecules and atoms and include the microscopic capillaries as well as the macroscopic genito-urinary tract, respiratory tract, lymphatics, veins, arteries and gastrointestinal tract.

Srotas carry digested food from the digestive tract to the basic tissue elements and provide nutrients for the formation of the seven *dhatus*. These include solids, liquids, gases, thought and nerve impulses, nutrients, waste products and secretions. This system of channels also carries the right proportions of the *doshas* (composed of the five great elements, see page 28) and the other basic tissue elements from one portion of the body to another. The *srota* system is also responsible for transporting the waste products to be eliminated via the *malas*.

This system is similar to the different physiological systems of Western medicine, but contains more subtle energy fields – much like the meridian system of Chinese medicine. In Western pathology diseases are classified according to the systems they involve, while in Ayurveda a complex symptomatology of channel-system disorders exists. Examination of the *srotas* through various diagnostic measures is one of the main tools for determining the nature, site and extent of disease.

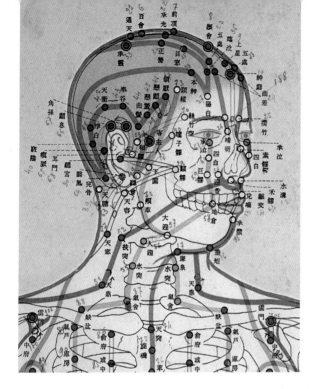

The srota *system is much like the meridian system of Chinese medicine.*

Disturbances

For proper functioning of a healthy body, the *srotas* must be open to allow free circulation of nutrients and other essential substances. If this is impaired or blocked for any reason, the circulating substance accumulates in the channels and metabolism of the tissue is affected. This gives rise to *Ama*, or toxins, which then circulates in the body through other channels that are still functioning. Excess *doshas* and *malas* can move into *srotas*. Blockage of the *srotas* is the beginning of disease.

There are four reasons for disturbance of the *srotas*:
1 Excessive flow: *Atipravurti*

2 Deficient flow/stagnation: *Sanga*

3 Blockage of the channels: *Shira granthi*

4 Disturbed/misdirected flow: *Vimarga gamana*

Vata governs all impulses and energy flow through the *srotas*, which are linked to the exterior – for instance, coughing, sneezing, crying, laughing, belching, passing wind, hiccoughing, urination and defecation. If these are suppressed, this can lead to disturbances in body and mind, such as anxiety, depression and unbalanced *gunas*. *Vata* is misdirected, which causes stagnation of wastes.

The 16 *srotas*

Charaka lists 13 *srotas* in his book, the Charaka Samhita: three for food, air and water, seven associated with the seven *dhatus* and three for excretion.

Presently there are 16 *srotas* identified.

Srotas that connect us with the outside environment

• *Prana vaha srota*: carries *Prana* (life force) through the respiratory system (the circulatory system and digestive system are also involved). *Prana* is absorbed through the lungs and colon and distributed with blood and plasma via the heart.

• *Anna vaha srota*: carries food (*anna*) mainly through the digestive system.

• *Ambhu or Udaka vaha srota*: carries water and regulates water metabolism; this includes the urinary tract and the fluid-absorbing aspect of the digestive tract. The origin is the palate and pancreas, which are involved in sugar metabolism.

Srotas that supply the seven *dhatus*

• *Rasa vaha srota*: carries plasma and lymphatic liquid

• *Rakta vaha srota*: carries blood through the circulatory system

• *Mamsa vaha srota*: carries

nutrients to the muscles and waste from muscle tissue
• *Meda vaha srota*: supplies fat to adipose tissues
• *Asthi vaha srota*: supplies nutrients to the bones

• *Majja vaha srota*: supplies nutrients to the bone marrow, nervous system and brain
• *Shukra vaha srota*: supplies nutrients to the sexual organs and carries reproductive cells and liquids

Srotas that allow for the elimination of wastes (*malas*)

• *Purisha vaha srota*: carries faeces
• *Mutra vaha srota*: carries urine
• *Sveda vaha srota*: carries sweat

Three additional *srotas* that are not described in the Charaka Samhita

• *Artava vaha srota* (the menstrual channel)
• *Stanya vaha srota* (the channel that carries breast milk)
• *Mano vaha srota* (the channel that carries all mental activities).

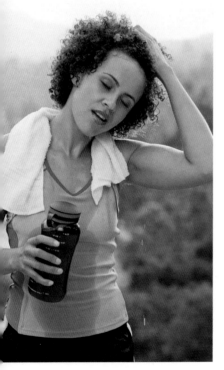

Sveda vaha srota *carries sweat, a pathway for the elimination of wastes.*

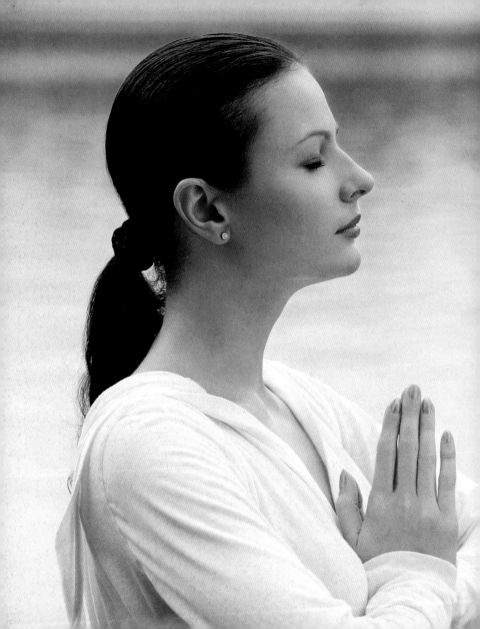

PART 2
MAINTAINING HEALTH AND WELL-BEING

Ayurveda is a complete way of life that encompasses guidance for each individual and their relationship to the world without and within them. This part of the book looks at how to assess your Ayurvedic constitution and explores the three *gunas,* the vital role of digestive fire and the six tastes.

Chapter 3: The three *gunas*

As we have seen, according to Ayurveda everything in creation is composed of three prime qualities or *gunas*, in varying proportions. These universal energies, known as *Sattva*, *Rajas* and *Tamas*, are attributed to the nature of the mind (*Manas*): *Sattva* as clarity, *Rajas* as action and *Tamas* as inertia.

Sattva, Rajas and *Tamas*

It is mainly on a mental level that the *gunas* have a significant effect. When in balance, they promote harmony and health. When *Rajas* or *Tamas* predominates, they can predispose to imbalance and ill health. We can clearly observe the effects of these qualities in the different mental and emotional states that we perennially experience.

Sattva is the quality of love, light, harmony, goodness and virtue. It promotes wisdom and intelligence, perception and clarity, joy and contentment. It enables spiritual awakening and development of the soul, and awakening of the five senses that enable us to experience the physical world around us. From *Sattva* comes the clarity or inner peace through which we can perceive the truth. Being *Sattvic* is the pure state to which many of us aspire. Health of mind and body is maintained by *Sattvic* living.

Rajas is the quality of energy, action and turbulence, which activates all movement, whether

From Sattva *comes the clarity or inner peace through which we can perceive the truth.*

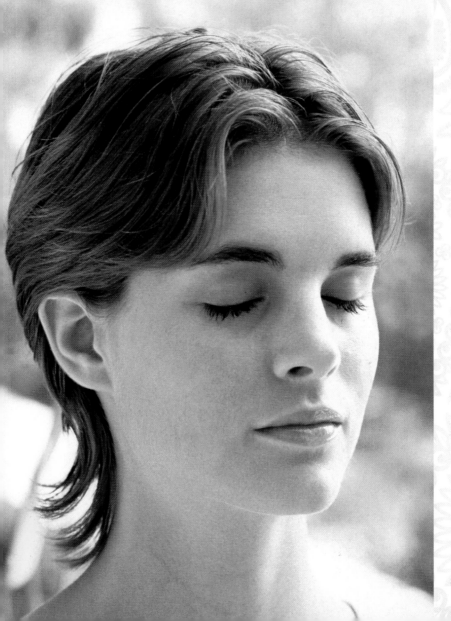

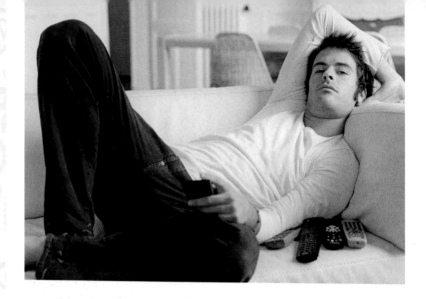

of ideas or instructions to the body. The three *doshas* ('humours' or life forces) – *Vata*, *Pitta* and *Kapha* – also arise primarily through *Rajas* as they are vital energies. In the mind *Rajas* provokes thought and is responsible for inspiration and creativity, but in excess it can cause restlessness, passion, aggression and overambition. It is said to give rise to self-motivated action that leads to pain and suffering, with a tendency to look for new stimuli, seeking fulfilment in the outer world. In a *Rajasic* state we can

Excess Tamas *can make us feel dull-minded and drowsy with little motivation.*

dissipate our energy through excess activity and, once we are tired and depressed, *Tamas* takes over.

Tamas is the quality of steadiness, dullness and inertia that causes sleep, decay, degeneration and death. Heavy and solid, it engenders calmness and steadiness – feeling 'as solid as a rock'. In the body it produces inactivity and sleep. An excess of *Tamas* in the mind can obstruct

86

movement, causing lethargy, attachment, irrationality, stubbornness, confusion, depression and delusion. We may feel dull-minded and drowsy, with little motivation; or struggle to see things clearly and be filled with doubts. Excess *Tamas* is responsible for ignorance and our inability to perceive our true inner selves.

Balancing the *gunas*

Although interaction of all three *gunas* is necessary, when *Sattva* predominates it makes for the correct balance. When *Sattva, Rajas* and *Tamas* act together in unity, this balance is known as 'pure *Sattva*', in which it is possible to quieten fluctuations of mood and cultivate a purer and more awakened mind. By eating a healthy *Sattvic* diet, and living a harmonious lifestyle with love, wisdom and other *Sattvic* attributes, we can experience inner peace and a sense of joy and fulfilment.

When *Rajas* or *Tamas* is excessive, this makes for ill health and unhappiness, and yet these *gunas* can still be seen positively. *Tamas* enables necessary relaxation and recovery from activity, so that we can replenish our energy. We need *Rajas* to survive in the world, for we cannot spend all day doing nothing in a *Sattvic* state of bliss! *Rajas* can also be used to convert *Tamas* into *Sattva*.

THE FIVE ELEMENTS AND THE THREE *GUNAS*

- *Akasha* (space) is represented in *Sattva*
- *Vayu* (air) and *Teja* (fire) are represented in *Rajas*
- *Prithvi* (earth) and *Jala* (water) are represented in *Tamas*

Foods and the *gunas*

In Ayurveda, food – like everything else in creation – falls into these same categories, and there are *Sattvic*, *Rajasic* and *Tamasic* foods, which have the ability to increase these qualities within us when we eat them.

Sattvic foods

Through *Sattvic* living we can help the nourishment of our bodies and promote the development of higher-quality tissues. *Sattvic* foods are considered to be the most healing, and also help to harmonize all three *doshas*.

These are the best-quality foods that enhance health and strength, energy and vitality, and lay the foundations for a *Sattvic* state of mind. These foods promote mental clarity, enhance love and compassion, and enable the development of a strong intellect and a good memory.

Sattvic foods are fresh, light, juicy, sweet, nourishing, energy-giving and tasty. They are full of

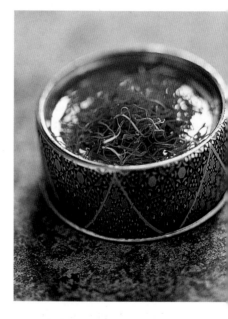

Sattvic *foods such as saffron are the most healing and help to harmonize all three* doshas.

Prana (life force) and are best eaten freshly prepared with love and in moderate amounts. They are easy to digest and therefore do not tax our energy through the process of digestion. *Sattvic* foods include:

• Most fresh organic vegetables, including carrots, sweet potatoes, parsnips, beetroot, turnips, salads, steamed leafy greens, asparagus, celery and cucumbers. Vegetables are best when lightly steamed (until crunchy-tender, not soft). Freshly made vegetable juices are rich in *Prana*, or live enzymes, and are easy to absorb.

• Most seasonal fruits and fruit juices, such as lemons, oranges, sweet apples, grapes, dates, bananas, figs, mangoes, pomegranates, peaches, pears, plums, prunes, apricots, cherries, blueberries and raspberries

• Coconut, coconut milk, cashews, hazelnuts, almonds, almond milk and butter, mung beans, chickpeas, lentils, sprouted beans, yellow split peas, aduki beans and organic tofu. To improve the digestibility of beans and pulses, soak them overnight, cook them with spices (such as asafoetida) or try sprouting them.

• Grains such as wheat, rye, buckwheat, barley, rice (particularly white basmati rice or long-grain brown rice), oats, quinoa and sprouted grain breads. Yeasted breads are not recommended unless they are toasted.

• Sunflower, pumpkin and sesame seeds and freshly ground flax seeds

• Raw cane sugar, maple syrup, agave nectar in small amounts and raw unheated honey

• Rock salt, black pepper, cinnamon, cardamom, cumin, coriander, fennel, fresh ginger and turmeric

• Freshly made unsweetened whole-milk yoghurt, lassi (see page 211), fresh milk (four hours after milking it becomes *Rajasic*), butter, ghee (clarified butter), unsweetened kefir (see page 211]) and homemade paneer (a curdled-milk cheese). Fresh, organic cow's milk is considered most *Sattvic* and is normally boiled before being consumed as this makes it more digestible. It is good lightly spiced (for example, with ginger, cinnamon or cardamom) and served with raw honey to overcome any mucus-forming tendencies. It should never be drunk cold straight from the fridge, or mixed with tastes that conflict with it, such as sour, pungent and salty ones, but should be taken alone or with other sweet-tasting foods like grains, sweet fruits and cereals. Avoid mixing yoghurt with fruit, as they are incompatible foods.

• Cold-pressed extra-virgin olive oil and sesame oil.

Rajasic foods

These are medium-quality foods, often high in protein and carbohydrate. They tend to be stimulating and capable of generating high levels of energy. They taste bitter, sour, salty and pungent, and have hot and dry qualities.

Rajasic foods include:
• Red and white meat, cheese, eggs and fish

• Garlic, onions, beans, the nightshade family (tomatoes, peppers, potatoes, aubergines), the brassica family (broccoli, cauliflower, cabbage, Brussels sprouts), radishes

• Hot, spicy and fried foods, especially chillies

• Sour, unripe fruits

• Pickles and chutneys

• Potatoes and other root vegetables

• Pasteurized milk

• Refined white sugar, carbonated drinks, sweets and biscuits

• Sea salt and salted bread

• Chocolate, caffeinated tea and coffee.

Sattvic foods become *Rajasic* if they are fried in oil and pungent spices, or overcooked. Foods that are hotter or colder than body temperature are also said to be *Rajasic*. We need *Rajasic* foods to enable us to carry out our activities and keep pace with the changing world, but excessive intake of them is said to create restlessness, excitement, agitation, anger, jealousy, deceit, egoism and over-high energy.

Tamasic foods

These are low-quality, devitalized foods and include unpalatable, overcooked, tinned, dried, processed, frozen and junk foods, as well as leftover food that has been 'spoiled' – that is, cooked and left too long to go off. *Tamasic* foods use a lot of energy in their digestion.

Tamasic foods include:

• Fizzy drinks and sweets

• Snacks such as crisps, chocolate, ice cream and popcorn

• Excessive alcohol and all intoxicants

• Foods containing additives and preservatives and all genetically modified foods

• Pork, beef, dark meats, onions, garlic, peanuts and dried milk

• Bread that is more than eight hours old

• Eggs and cheeses

• Mushrooms and avocados

• Fried and fermented foods, vinegar

• Overripe fruit and vegetables
• Overcooked, frozen, canned, boxed and microwaved foods, leftovers and reheated foods.

Hot and cold foods taken together, and incompatible food combinations such as milk and vinegar, radishes and honey, bread and bananas, produce *Tamas*.

Overeating in general, and eating snacks late in the evening, also increase *Tamas*. *Tamasic* foods are best avoided as much as possible. In children they are said to predispose to behavioural problems like hyperactivity.

To make the best of our predominantly *Sattvic* diet it is best to eat slowly and in moderate amounts. The general Ayurvedic guidelines are to eat until you are three-quarters full, leaving quarter of your stomach empty to allow room for your digestive enzymes to mix properly with your food.

AYURVEDIC FOODS AT A GLANCE

	Sattvic	*Rajasic*	*Tamasic*
Grains	Rice, tapioca, rye, wheat, blue corn, barley, rice milk	Millet, buckwheat, corn	
Nuts and seeds	Nuts, seeds and nut mixes		
Fruit	Pears, peaches, figs, bananas, pomegranates, oranges, plums, lemons, grapes, dates	Apples, guavas, sour fruits	Avocados, water-melons, apricots

	Sattvic	*Rajasic*	*Tamasic*
Vegetables	Carrots, sweet potatoes, beetroot, lettuce, sprouts	Potatoes, tomatoes, cauliflower, onions, broccoli, spinach, garlic	Mushrooms
Beans and pulses		Aduki beans, toor dhal	Black beans, pinto beans, urad dhal
Herbs and spices	Anise, cardamom, coriander, turmeric, cumin, fennel, fenugreek seeds, rose, saffron, flax seeds	Chillies, asafoetida, bay leaves, black pepper, cinnamon, cloves, fenugreek leaves, ginger, mint	
Meat and fish		Fish, shrimps, chicken	Beef, lamb, pork
Condiments	Rock salt	Sea salt	
Sweeteners	Honey, raw cane sugar	Sugar (refined)	White sugar
Dairy products	Fresh milk, fresh yoghurt, lassi, butter, ghee	Eggs, sour milk, homogenized milk, sour cream	Hard cheese
Other foods		Fried food, salted bread, sweets, biscuits, salted crisps, chips, pickles, chutneys, tea, coffee, alcohol	Old stale food, preservatives, overcooked food, frozen food, dried food, fizzy drinks, peanuts, sweets, crisps, ice cream, popcorn, alcohol

Chapter 4: **Assessing your Ayurvedic constitution**

According to Ayurveda, the key to health lies in the knowledge and understanding of our basic constitution (*Prakruti*) and how to keep it in balance through diet and lifestyle. If we don't live according to the needs of our individual constitution, the *doshas* ('humours') will become unbalanced and lead to ill health (*Vyadhi*).

With the knowledge and understanding of how and why we become ill, we can live a way of life that maximizes our chances of health and fulfilment. The Ayurvedic system provides details of the right foods and drinks for each constitution: whether they should be cold or hot, raw or cooked; which tastes they should have; which herbs and spices should be taken regularly; which is the best form of exercise; which time of year is best and when more care needs to be taken; when is the best time to wake up, and when to go to bed.

Ayurveda is a complete way of life that encompasses guidance for the individual and their relationship to the world without and within them.

Ayurveda advises about the right foods and drink for each constitution.

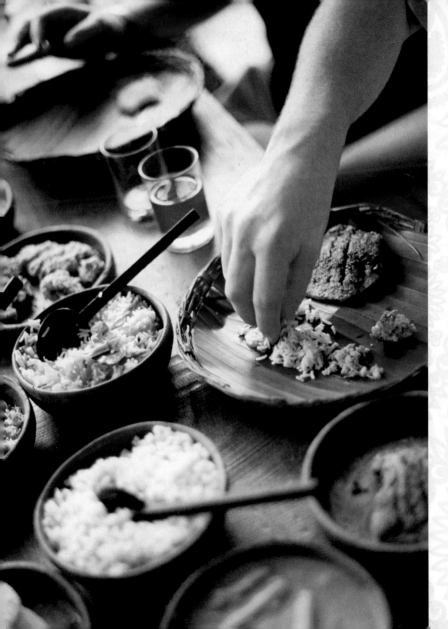

Prakruti and *Vikruti*

We are all composed of varying proportions of the three *doshas*, *Vata*, *Pitta* and *Kapha*. Between them the *doshas* are responsible for all activity in mind and body, including our digestion, the metabolism of all our cells and tissues, our thoughts and feelings, our health and our predisposition to disease.

We are born with our own individual balance of *doshas*, which is brought about mainly by the *dosha* balance in our parents at the time of our conception. This is our basic constitution (*Prakruti*) and it remains unchanged throughout our lives. *Prakruti* actually means 'nature', 'creativity' or 'the first creation'. Factors that govern our *Prakruti* include:

- The condition of sperm and ovum, known as *Sukra-Shonit Prakruti*
- The condition of the uterus, called *Kala-garbhasaya Prakruti*
- The diet followed by the mother during pregnancy, known as *Matu-ahar Prakruti*.

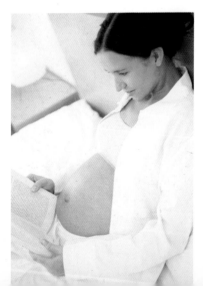

The diet followed by our mothers during pregnancy influences our Prakruti.

Our individual characteristics

The dominant *dosha* (or *doshas*) in our *Prakruti* determines our body type, our temperament and the health problems to which we may be susceptible. Our *Prakruti* is our gift for life, the incarnation in which we can travel further toward enlightenment, and it makes us the unique individual we are – different in material and subtle ways from anyone else in the universe, down to our DNA and our fingerprints. The concept of *Prakruti* provides a reasonable explanation for the fact that two people can react very differently when exposed to the same environment, food or stimuli. Thus, in order to understand others and ourselves, it is necessary to determine our *Prakruti*.

In order to keep our *doshas* in balance, through the right diet and lifestyle, it is first of all important to determine exactly what our *Prakruti* is. If it is disturbed by diet, lifestyle, experience or state of mind, for example, the disruption may be felt as physical discomfort and pain, or as mental and emotional suffering, such as fear and anxiety, anger or jealousy. Our current state of imbalance of the *doshas* causing such symptoms is known as our *Vikruti*.

Our *Vikruti* reflects our dynamic homeostatic mechanisms, which are constantly adjusting to the influences of life inside and outside us, and so it is always changing. Ideally the *doshic* balance of our *Vikruti* should match our *Prakruti* as closely as possible. The purpose of Ayurvedic treatment is to return the *doshic* balance of our *Vikruti* to that of our *Prakruti*.

Determining our constitution

One or two (or, rarely, three) of the *doshas* will dominate in our constitution. Single-*doshic* types are the easiest to determine, because one *dosha* stands out more clearly than the other two. *Vata*

DETERMINING YOUR CONSTITUTION

There are basically seven different *Prakrutis*:

1 V = predominantly *Vata*

2 P = predominantly *Pitta*

3 K = predominantly *Kapha*

4 VP or PV = equal *Vata* and *Pitta* (perhaps one *dosha* slightly more than the other)

5 VK or KV = equal *Vata* and *Kapha*

6 PK or KP = equal *Pitta* and *Kapha*

7 VPK = all three *doshas* equal

types tend to be slim and small-boned, often with irregular shapes or facial features. They feel cold and have dry skin, and are often highly creative, restless, unpredictable and energetic, and yet tire easily (see page 36). *Pitta* types have a medium, athletic build, well-proportioned with sharp facial features. They are dynamic, ambitious, competitive and passionate, and tend to feel hot and sensitive, both physically and emotionally (see page 42).

Kapha types have a larger build, heavy bones and tend put on weight easily as they have a slow metabolism. They are strong, resilient, grounded, calm, routine-oriented, loyal and dependable. They have thick skin, which ages well, thick hair and strong teeth (see page 48).

Many of us exhibit more than one of the *dosha* characteristics. It is important to understand that we all have the three *doshas*. For many people two of the three *doshas* can exist in a higher proportion relative to the third. These are mixed-*dosha* types. It is quite common, for example, to be a *Pitta-Kapha* type exhibiting physical and emotional characteristics of both *doshas*. A small percentage of people will actually have equal proportions of all three, making them *tridosha* types.

Diagnosing *Prakruti* and *Vikruti*

Both *Prakruti* and *Vikruti* can be ascertained by careful diagnosis, which involves taking a detailed case history and examining the body, paying attention to build, skin and hair type, the temperature of the body, digestion and bowel function. In the case of arthritis,

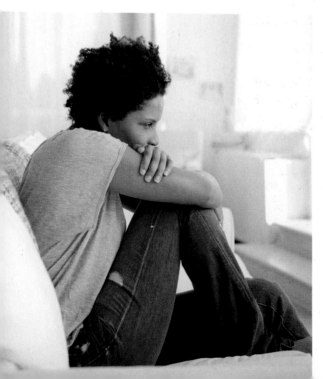

Kapha types are strong, grounded and love relaxing.

we can accumulate toxins in the system due to poor diet, weak digestion, stress and a sedentary lifestyle. These can then circulate and settle in the joints, and the way this manifests as symptoms varies according to the *doshas* involved. *Vata* type is a dry, degenerative kind of arthritis, with sharp, erratic pain and dry, cracking joints accompanied by anxiety and possibly bloating and wind. A *Pitta* type is more inflammatory with burning pain and hot, swollen joints and irritability. *Kapha* type involves dull, aching pain and large, watery, swollen joints and lethargy.

Pulse and tongue diagnosis are valuable tools for confirming an analysis of health and constitution. In these respects Ayurveda has much in common with Chinese and Tibetan medicine, in which these two indicators of someone's state of health are also very important. A highly complex technique for taking the patient's pulse has been developed by Ayurvedic practitioners, which requires many years of practice to perfect (see page 173).

Once you know your *Prakruti* and *Vikruti* you will understand much more about yourself and why you react the way you do and are prone to certain health problems. This will enable you to choose more precisely the right diet and correct lifestyle advice for your *doshas*, and you can then implement specific treatment. The first step back to health is the elimination of toxins and enhancing your digestion or raising digestive fire (*Agni*) (see page 214).

To illustrate, a health problem associated with excess *Kapha* could be characterized by catarrh, lethargy, being overweight and fluid retention. A diet consisting of warm, dry, light food would be advised, since *Kapha* is cool and damp. Avoidance of foods with a cold, damp quality – such as wheat, milk products and sugar – which would serve to increase *Kapha* would also be recommended. Herbal remedies would include

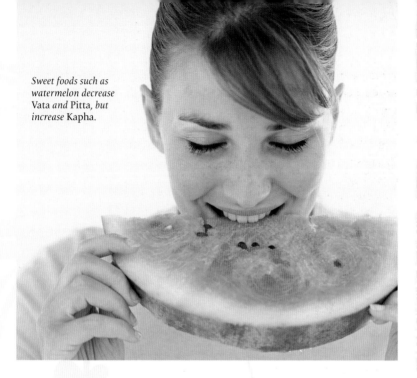

Sweet foods such as watermelon decrease Vata *and* Pitta, *but increase* Kapha.

warming spices like ginger, cinnamon, cloves and pepper to raise digestive fire and cleanse toxins from the body. Bitters such as turmeric and aloe vera may also be prescribed. The specific choice of herbal remedy depends on its 'quality' or 'energy', which Ayurveda determines according to 20 attributes (see page 76), such as hot, cold, wet, dry, heavy or light.

Ayurveda also classifies remedies according to six tastes: sweet, sour, salty, pungent, bitter and astringent. Sweet, sour and salty substances increase *Kapha* and decrease *Vata*; pungent, bitter and astringent tastes decrease *Kapha* and increase *Vata*; while sweet, bitter and astringent tastes decrease *Pitta* and pungent, salty and sour tastes increase *Pitta*.

Questionnaire: determine your *Prakruti* and *Vikruti*

Complete the checklist on pages 101–105. Using a coloured pen, tick the box (or boxes) in each row with the attributes that most closely resemble those you have had for most of your life, going back to your earliest memories (you may need to consult your family for details that you do not clearly remember). This will determine your *Prakruti*. Then go through the questions again and, using a different-coloured pen, tick the box (or boxes) that most closely resemble your *present* state. This will help determine your *Vikruti*.

Add up all the ticks for the different *doshas* in one colour, to determine your *Prakruti* (e.g. 22 *Vata*, 12 *Pitta*, 16 *Kapha*). Then add up all the ticks in the other colour to determine your *Vikruti* (e.g. 27 *Vata*, 10 *Pitta*, 8 *Kapha*). *In this example* Vata *has increased, meaning that there is a* Vata *imbalance.*

QUESTIONNAIRE

Characteristic	*Vata* attribute	*Pitta* attribute	*Kapha* attribute
Weight	☐ below average ☐ loses weight easily	☐ medium weight ☐ concerned about maintaining the right weight	☐ heavy ☐ gains weight easily
Body frame	☐ small-boned	☐ medium-boned	☐ large-boned
Muscles	☐ undeveloped	☐ well developed	☐ solid/flabby
Height	☐ below or above average	☐ medium height	☐ average to tall
Hips	☐ narrow	☐ medium	☐ wide
Hair	☐ dry, brittle, thin ☐ curly/coarse ☐ dark	☐ fine, straight, oily ☐ blond, red ☐ early balding/greying	☐ thick, oily ☐ curly/lustrous ☐ dark
Body hair	☐ scanty	☐ moderate	☐ thick
Face	☐ irregular features	☐ prominent features	☐ rounded
Eyes	☐ small, nervous ☐ dry	☐ medium, penetrating red, sensitive to smoke/bright light	☐ large, moist, thick eyelashes ☐ calm and gentle
Nose	☐ small ☐ long, bent	☐ medium ☐ straight, pointed	☐ large ☐ wide

QUESTIONNAIRE

Characteristic	*Vata* attribute	*Pitta* attribute	*Kapha* attribute
Lips	☐ small ☐ dark	☐ medium ☐ soft, red	☐ large ☐ velvety
Skin	☐ rough, dry ☐ cold, thin ☐ tans easily ☐ dark	☐ oily, warm, moist ☐ delicate, sensitive, burns easily, freckles/moles ☐ radiant, glowing ☐ reddish/yellowish	☐ soft and smooth ☐ cool and oily ☐ thick and pale ☐ tends to burn
Temperature	☐ dislikes cold, windy, dry weather ☐ loves heat ☐ perspiration is scanty with no smell	☐ dislikes heat and strong sun ☐ loves winter ☐ perspires easily with strong smell	☐ comfortable in most weathers ☐ dislikes cold and damp ☐ perspires moderately with pleasant smell
Nails	☐ brittle, dry ☐ ridged	☐ well formed ☐ soft	☐ strong, thick ☐ smooth
Hands and feet	☐ cold, dry	☐ warm, moist, pink	☐ cool, damp
Body fat	☐ around the hips and thighs	☐ evenly distributed ☐ round the waist	☐ around the thighs and buttocks

QUESTIONNAIRE

Characteristic	*Vata* attribute	*Pitta* attribute	*Kapha* attribute
Energy level	☐ very active, comes in spurts ☐ low endurance, tires easily	☐ active, determined, ☐ can push themselves to work long hours	☐ strong, but lethargic ☐ once motivated, endurance is good
Movement	☐ fast	☐ medium	☐ slow and steady
Mental attitude	☐ flexible, adaptable ☐ restless, changeable ☐ quick, indecisive	☐ ambitious, competitive ☐ practical, organized, efficient ☐ intense, discriminating	☐ calm, peaceful ☐ dull ☐ slow, methodical ☐ patient
Way of learning	☐ takes things in quickly ☐ learns through listening ☐ enjoys doing lots of things at once ☐ can lose focus	☐ analyses and digests material easily ☐ learns through reading/visual aids ☐ focused and discriminating, finishes what they start	☐ takes things in slowly ☐ retains information ☐ may learn through association, methodical
Emotional attitude	☐ lively ☐ intuitive ☐ anxious, fearful, insecure ☐ changeable ☐ talks about their feelings	☐ perceptive ☐ irritable, prone to anger ☐ intolerant, aggressive ☐ keeps feelings to themselves	☐ resilient ☐ loyal, stable, dependable ☐ compassionate, nurturing ☐ clingy ☐ complacent, in denial

QUESTIONNAIRE

Characteristic	Vata attribute	Pitta attribute	Kapha attribute
Memory	☐ good short-term ☐ quick to grasp ☐ quick to forget	☐ good medium-term ☐ distinct ☐ clear	☐ good long-term ☐ slow to grasp ☐ never forgets
Speech	☐ fast, talkative ☐ imaginative ☐ interrupted, chaotic	☐ sharp ☐ convincing ☐ clear, detailed, precise	☐ slow, steady ☐ melodious, soothing ☐ could be dull
Creativity	☐ inventive, rich in ideas ☐ good at starting, but doesn't complete projects	☐ inventive, technical ☐ gets things done	☐ methodical, ☐ business-minded
Sleep	☐ light, easily interrupted ☐ irregular, 5–6 hours	☐ short and even ☐ 6–8 hours	☐ long and deep ☐ over 8 hours, hard to wake up
Dreams	☐ active, frightening ☐ running, flying	☐ passionate, fiery, angry, violent ☐ the sun	☐ gentle, romantic, sentimental ☐ water
Eating habits	☐ irregular	☐ regular, eats frequently due to tendency to hypoglycaemia	☐ eats large amounts, but can go for long periods between eating

QUESTIONNAIRE

Characteristic	Vata attribute	Pitta attribute	Kapha attribute
Appetite	☐ variable, skips meals	☐ strong, cannot miss meals	☐ low, but loves food and can be greedy
Bowels	☐ dry, hard, rabbit droppings	☐ soft, oily, loose stools	☐ heavy, slow, large stools
Sensitive to	☐ noise	☐ bright light	☐ smells
Spending habits	☐ doesn't save ☐ spends money on trifles	☐ moderate saver ☐ spends money on luxuries	☐ thrifty, accumulates wealth ☐ spends money on food
Hobbies	☐ travelling ☐ art, music, going out ☐ philosophy, esoteric subjects	☐ sports, keeping fit ☐ debating, politics ☐ luxury, style, looking good	☐ relaxing ☐ staying at home ☐ good food
Sex drive	☐ changeable, high or low ☐ can be intense	☐ moderate ☐ passionate, can be controlling	☐ slow to arouse ☐ loyal and devoted
Pulse	☐ thready, moves like a snake ☐ fast and irregular	☐ strong, jumps like a frog ☐ regular	☐ deep, glides like a swan ☐ slow and regular

Chapter 5: *Agni* – the vital role of digestive fire

Our health largely depends on how well we are able to digest, absorb and utilize the nutrients from our food. While food conversion provides energy, it also requires energy to perform all the essential biochemical reactions involved in the process. If the digestive energy is weak or disturbed, stomach aches, diarrhoea or constipation may arise, as well as more generalized symptoms such as lethargy, headaches, irritability, poor concentration, disturbed sleep and lowered immunity.

Optimal functioning of the digestive tract depends on several factors. First, regular peristaltic (wave-like) movements require sufficient dietary fibre to push food through the gut, so that we can evacuate food residues as well as the waste products of metabolism. Poor elimination leads to a toxic state of the bowel, which then becomes prone to infection and spreads toxins to the rest of the body.

Second, there is constant interaction between the brain and the digestive tract, making digestion highly susceptible to the effects of mind and emotion, personality and constitution. Stress can, for example, reduce the flow of digestive enzymes and thereby reduce digestion and absorption; or cause excess hydrochloric acid in the stomach, irritating the stomach or intestine linings.

Our ability to digest is like a fire that transforms the food we eat into tiny molecules that we can absorb.

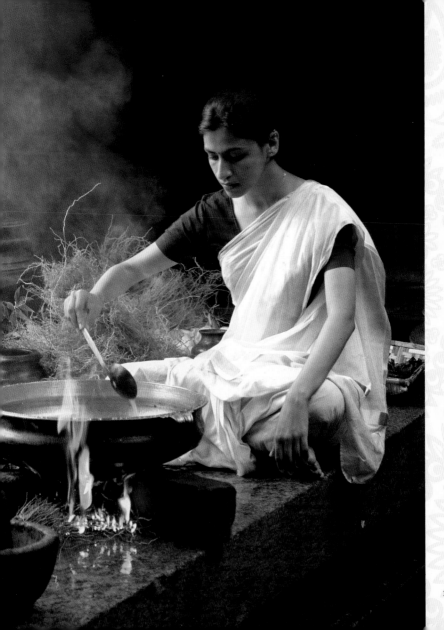

The Ayurvedic approach to digestion

Just as our bodies are made up of the five elements – earth, water, fire, air and ether – so is the food we eat. Our appetite and our ability to digest and absorb nutrients with the help of digestive enzymes is known as *Agni* or 'digestive fire', and this is central to health.

Agni is a Vedic term meaning 'burning, transforming, or perceiving', from the root *ang*, meaning 'to burst forth'. Our *Agni*, or digestive power, enables our bodies to utilize the five elements in food, extract the nutrients and transform them into bodily elements.

In its broadest sense *Agni* is the fire that transforms all food, as well as sensations coming into the body, into energy and enables us to absorb them as nourishment for our tissues. We digest all that we eat, see, hear, smell, touch and taste. And our digestive fire plays the central role.

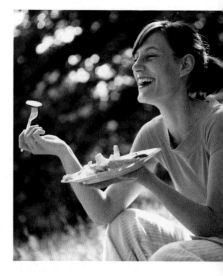

We digest and absorb our food with the help of digestive enzymes known as Agni, *or digestive fire.*

THE 13 FORMS OF *AGNI*

There are many different types of fire in the body, the main form of which is digestive fire.

- *Jatharagni*: This is the digestive fire that imparts energy to all the secretions and enzymes in the process of digestion, and resides in the stomach and small intestine. It is responsible not simply for digesting and absorbing nutrients from food, but also for destroying pathogenic (disease-causing) microorganisms in the gut. If the digestive fire is low and digestion incomplete as a result, partially digested or undigested food ferments and breeds toxins in the gut, thereby compromising the immune system.

- **5 elemental fires, or *Bhutagnis*:** Each of the five elements has its own digestive fire. These reside in the liver, and are responsible for turning digestive fire into *Agni* that corresponds to each of the five elements, essential for building up the respective tissues in the body. If their functioning is impaired, the relevant element in the body will not be formed correctly. Substances such as ghee or aloe-vera gel help to regulate elemental digestive fires.

- **7 tissue fires, or *Dhatuagnis*:** Each of the 7 *dhatus* (tissues) has its own digestive fire, responsible for proper formation of that tissue. When *Agni* is too low, too much tissue of an inferior nature will be formed. When it is too high, insufficient tissue will be formed (see page 64).

According to Ayurveda, when *Agni* is sufficient, it prevents the build-up of toxins in the body; the mind and senses are clear and acute; and we have the energy to channel our lives in a positive direction. When deficient, it causes a build-up of toxins (*Ama*) in the body, which gives rise to dullness, heaviness, stagnation and cloudiness of mind and perception.

Elemental *Agnis*

Digestive fire works on the food mass that has been swallowed and liquefied. It separates the pure or nutritive part of the food (*sara*) from the waste material (*kitta*) and breaks it down into the five elements. These in turn are absorbed and transferred to the liver, where the elemental *Agnis* turn them into the respective elemental tissues (*dhatus*) for the body:

- The earth elements that are digested and transformed from the food serve to build up the basic bulk or protein of the body, like the muscles
- The water element builds up the vital fluids, plasma, blood and fat
- The fire elements build up the enzymes and haemoglobin
- The air elements build up bone and nerves
- The ether elements build up the mind and senses.

Prana Vata (see page 54) helps in the digestion of food. *Samana Vata* (see page 55) controls peristaltic movements and the absorption of food. *Apana Vata* (see page 56) controls defecation and the expulsion of gases.

Stages of digestion

According to Ayurveda there are three stages of digestion governed by the *doshas*):

1 The first stage is governed by *Kapha* and takes place in the mouth and stomach. It involves saliva and the alkaline secretions of the stomach, and is responsible for the extraction of the water and earth elements from the food that

Eating too many light and dry foods will aggravate Vata.

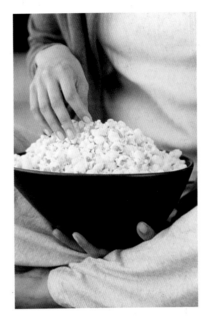

is eaten. *Kapha*-predominant people tend to have an excess of these secretions and are prone to symptoms such as nausea, mucus, profuse salivation and poor appetite, especially if they eat too many sweet and salty foods.

2 The second stage is ruled by *Pitta* and involves the acid secretions from the stomach and small intestine. Here the fire element is extracted from our food. Eating too many sour, salty and pungent foods can increase these secretions and give rise to heartburn, indigestion, burning stomach pains, nausea and diarrhoea.

3 The third stage is ruled by *Vata*, and takes place in the large intestine and involves the reabsorption of water and formation of stools. Here the air and ether elements are extracted from foods. Eating too many light, dry, astringent, bitter or pungent foods or too many hard, raw foods, including salads, will increase *Vata* and give rise to symptoms such as wind, bloating, abdominal pain and constipation. Too many raw foods, salads and hard, dry nuts and seeds may also aggravate *Vata*.

Looking after your *Agni*

Maintaining the equilibrium of the digestive fire is the key to preventative health, as well as to the treatment of most problems. A fire has to be kept stoked and provided with the right fuel so that it does not go out. It can burn too low or rage too high. Balance is the key to good digestion.

We can compare our *Agni* to the sun. In the morning, when it first comes up, it is not very hot as we have been sleeping and fasting all night. We need to stoke the fire, in the shape of a hot cup of freshly grated ginger tea or hot water with a squeeze of fresh lemon or lime juice. Then we can follow it with a light breakfast. At midday the sun is at its hottest, and our *Agni* is at its strongest and burning well enough to take a good-sized meal. By evening, as the sun sets, our energy and digestion begin to slow down again and our *Agni* is lower. This is the time to eat another light meal and then rest and relax. We don't need so much fuel for evening activities, and if we put heavy logs on the fire they will not burn properly and could disturb our digestion or our sleep. Our bodies do not need the energy or fuel that they did earlier. In addition:

• **Don't eat more than you need**. Smaller, lighter meals are better than large, heavy ones, which can overload the fire and put it out! According to Ayurveda, we should eat until our stomach feels three-quarters full and then leave one-quarter of the space to enable our digestive juices to mix properly with our food and thus optimize digestion.

• **Taste and enjoy your food**. Eating food you dislike will inhibit the flow of digestive enzymes. Eating with awareness will promote good digestion.

• **Eat slowly and in a relaxed fashion, sitting down**. Digestive enzymes flow when the parasympathetic nervous system is in operation. When adrenaline flows, our digestive enzymes don't.

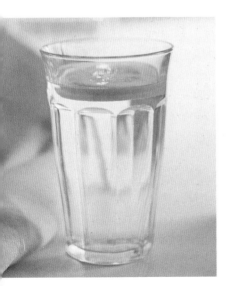

So it is important to be relaxed and not to eat on the run.

• **When you eat, only eat**. When you eat consciously, and taste your food, your body is more likely to secrete the appropriate digestive juices to digest the food being eaten. If you are watching TV (especially if the programme produces stress), working at your computer or discussing something inflammatory such as religion, politics or your relationship, this is likely to disturb your digestion. Light, relaxed conversation with friends or family is fine.

•**Sit quietly before eating, to let go of any stress**. Saying grace is a good way to do this.

• **Drink some hot water with fresh lemon** or lime juice, or freshly grated ginger, to kindle your digestion before a meal.

Hot water with fresh lemon juice first thing in the morning will help stoke your digestive fire.

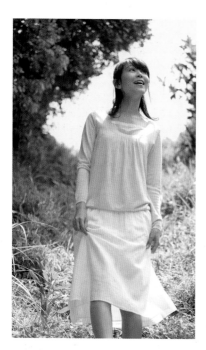

A gentle walk after a meal will help promote good digestion.

cumin, coriander and fennel. You can also drink them in teas.

• **Eat when you feel hungry** and once your previous meal has been digested, preferably allowing at least four hours between meals. Grazing or snacking is not great for the digestion. If you have high *Agni*, however, you may need to eat more often than this to prevent low blood sugar.

• **Don't eat late**. Allow two to three hours after your evening meal before going to bed. Going to sleep on a full stomach is not advisable. You will feel much better in the morning if you eat a light meal around at around 6 or 7 p.m.

• **Don't drink too much with your meals**.

• **Go for a gentle walk after you eat**, to promote digestion and settle your food.

• **Add mild spices to your cooking**, such as turmeric, ginger,

• **Do not fast or skip meals** unless you are undergoing a detoxification programme.

• **Eat regularly and at the same time every day**, so that your *Agni* can prepare for the meal.

The four conditions of *Agni*

There are four different conditions of *Agni* – variable (*Visham*), high (*Tikshna*), low (*Manda*) and balanced (*Sama*), each of which has different effects on the body.

Variable *Agni* (*Vishamagni*)

Digestive fire tends to be variable in *Vata* types, with their fluctuating nature and nervous digestion. It is caused by over-heavy/light diet and activities that increase *Vata*, and in turn it causes *Vata*-type disorders. If your *Agni* is variable, you can be alternately very hungry and not hungry at all, and sometimes you will digest well and at other times

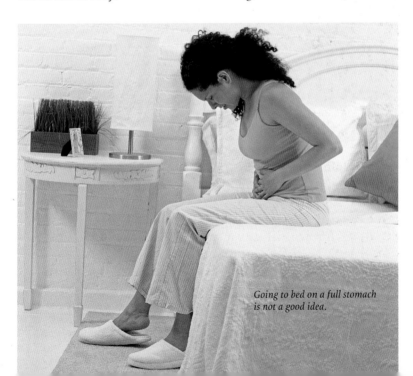

Going to bed on a full stomach is not a good idea.

you may suffer from: bloating and wind, constipation, diarrhoea, irritable bowel syndrome or discomfort in the abdomen, borborygmi (rumblings in the gut) or colicky pain. After a while *Vishamagni* becomes low digestive fire and the ability to digest well diminishes.

High *Agni* (*Tikshnagni*)

Digestive fire is usually high in *Pitta* types, who generally have a good appetite and digestion without gaining excessive weight. *Agni* can be overly increased by eating hot, spicy food in hot weather, and by activities that increase *Pitta,* and in turn it disrupts digestive enzymes and causes *Pitta*-type disorders. If *Agni* is too high you will want to eat more, you digest quickly, your metabolic rate is fast and you may be prone to: indigestion, belching, nausea, acidity, low blood sugar (causing weakness, irritability or headaches), stomach aches, gastritis, peptic ulcers, fevers or diarrhoea. Eventually the fire burns itself out,

often through diarrhoea or infection, and results in low digestive fire.

Low *Agni* (*Mandagni*)

Agni is usually low in *Kapha* types who have a slow metabolism and a tendency to hold weight, even without eating excessively. *Mandagni* is caused by diet and activities that increase *Kapha,* including eating too much heavy, indigestible, oily and sweet foods, such as cheese (not ghee), eating stale or cold foods and cold drinks, drinking too much liquid with meals, a sedentary lifestyle and excessive sleep. It can also be the result of disturbance to the digestion from eating irregularly, excessive fasting, stress and high *Vata,* and from debility and illness such as gastroenteritis and chronic diarrhoea. Low digestive fire leads to *Kapha* disorders such as: mucus congestion, a tendency to frequent colds and coughs, slow digestion, sluggish bowels, a feeling of dullness, heaviness in the stomach,

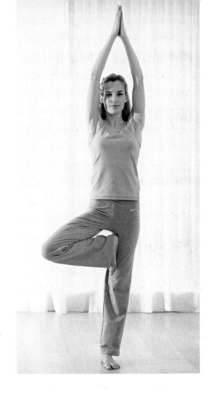

Good Agni *can be maintained by regular exercise, such as yoga, and deep breathing (*Pranayama*).*

a tendency to coughs and breathlessness, lethargy or a feeling of heaviness in the body, sleepiness after eating, excess saliva or nausea. Symptoms are worse with *Ama* (toxins) causing joint pain, headache, sinusitis and lassitude.

Balanced *Agni* (*Samagni*)

Digestive fire is balanced when the *doshas* and emotions are in harmony. It is indicated by a regular and moderate appetite, with efficient digestion promoting good health. People with *Samagni* can tolerate hunger, heavy food and irregular or excessive food intake and still preserve good digestive fire. When *Agni* is normal, mild *Sattvic* spices such as cardamom, turmeric, coriander and fennel can be taken through diet to maintain the health of the digestive tract. *Agni* can also be maintained by regular exercise, yoga, deep breathing (*Pranayama*), meditation and proper eating. Ill health develops as a result of excess, deficient or abnormal *Agni*, which eventually becomes low digestive fire. Weak *Agni* lowers immunity, as *Ama* (undigested food mass) is formed from poor digestion and obstructs the channels (*srotas*) throughout the body.

TREATMENT FOR DISTURBANCES OF *AGNI*

Treatment for *Vishamagni: Vata shamana*

Oily (e.g. ghee), mild spicy, sour and salty foods and medicines help to balance digestive fire when combined with a light diet. Useful formulae (see Chapter 16) include: Hingwashtaka Churna, Lavanbhaskar Churna (1/8 to ¼ teaspoon with warm ghee before meals, see page 345) and Lashunadi Vati.

Vehicle to carry herbs to the tissues (*Anupana*): warm water/ghee

Treatment for *Tikshnagni: Pitta shamana*

Hot spices should be avoided and digestive bitters such as chamomile, guduchi, dandelion root, rosemary and amalaki with their cooling properties can be taken. Heavy, cold, unctuous and sweet foods are useful. Laxatives can be taken once every two to four weeks, such as Triphala or Darthree. Coriander, amalaki and shatavari cool Pitta. Mahasudarshan Churna lowers digestive fire without increasing toxins.

Vehicle (*Anupana*): cool water/ghee

Treatment for *Mandagni: Kapha shamana*

If you have low *Agni*, foods will not be digested easily and the stomach will be upset by a number of foods or combinations of foods. Food intolerances and allergies may develop. You can enhance the digestion by using herbs and eating easily digested foods in moderate (rather than large) meals. Red meats, cheese and raw foods are best avoided as they are hard to digest, especially in the evenings. Excess milk products and foods containing sugar are also best avoided. Warm foods are more easily digested than cold, raw, hard foods, so soups, stews and casseroles are better than salads.

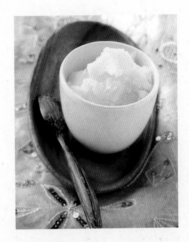

Ghee is highly regarded in Ayurveda. It enhances digestion, helps clear toxins and increases Ojas.

Appetizing, digestive, bitter, pungent and astringent foods and medicines are given to stimulate *Agni*. Spices are particularly good, and the following formulae and herbs are indicated: Trikatu, cayenne, ginger, pippali, chitrak, musta, guduchi, bilva fruit and asafoetida.

Spices also digest *Ama*, while astringent, bitter and pungent herbs dry excess liquid or mucus, which can dampen digestive fire. Hingwashtaka Churna, Trikatu and ginger are effective *Ama*-reducing remedies.

The undigested food mass (*Ama*)

If your digestive fire is low, it leaves a residue of undigested or partly digested food that can accumulate, stagnate and ferment in the gut, feeding pathogenic microorganisms and causing dysbiosis (the disturbance of the normal gut flora). This is known as *Ama*.

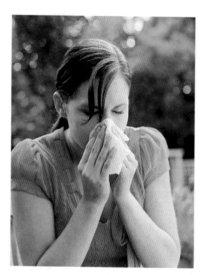

Ama undermines our defence system and lowers immunity, predisposing us to the common cold.

Once *Ama* is absorbed into the body, it obstructs normal functioning of the tissues and weakens our immune systems. It undermines our defence system and lowers resistance to disease, starting with the common cold. It tends to affect areas of weakness and underlies symptoms in both body and mind, such as lowered energy, anxiety and depression. Hence *Agni* is the key to health.

Intestinal bacteria

The intestinal bacteria in a healthy gut play a very important role in our general health. They synthesize vitamins, including vitamin B; aid

SYMPTOMS OF *AMA*

- Poor appetite, indigestion and bowel problems
- Bloating, smelly wind or stools, undigested food in the faeces
- Allergic reactions, such as asthma, hives, psoriasis and eczema
- Mental and physical fatigue, sleepiness or heaviness after eating
- Bad breath and body odour
- Lethargy and depression, low enthusiasm and motivation, lack of mental clarity
- Waking up tired, even after a good night's sleep
- Lack of lustre in the eyes and skin
- Skin problems
- White/cream coating on the tongue, particularly noticeable in the morning
- Aches and pains
- Headaches and migraine
- Recurrent infections
- Congestion causing constipation, catarrh and vaginal thrush
- Emotional instability, short attention span and behavioural problems in children
- Raised cholesterol and atherosclerosis (plaque in the arteries)

the absorption of minerals and trace elements, including calcium and magnesium; break down dietary toxins, making them less harmful; stimulate local immunity (inhibiting infections such as *Salmonella*, decreasing the risk of food poisoning); and enhance general immunity. In fact four-fifths of the body's immune system is found in the gut lining.

Poor digestion, the fermentation of undigested foods and stress disturb the balance of the intestinal flora. This is aggravated by the use of antibiotics and steroids and leads to the proliferation of pathogenic yeasts and bacteria in our intestines. These create toxins, destroy vitamins, inactivate digestive enzymes and lead to the formation of chemicals that are potentially carcinogenic (cancer-causing). They provoke inflammatory diseases, including ulcerative colitis and Crohn's disease by causing leaky gut syndrome and autoimmune reactions, as well as liver problems.

Clearing *Ama*

Ayurveda explains clearly how to remedy the situation if you show evidence of *Ama*. You need to strengthen your digestion and clear any toxins. Your dietary guidelines are determined by the balance of your *doshas* and the state of your *Agni*, but generally speaking you can do the following:

• Eat regularly. Don't miss meals.
• Eat a light, fresh, healthy diet.
• Avoid high-*Kapha* foods because *Ama* is heavy, sticky and has the ability to get stuck, just like *Kapha*. Avoid overeating and don't eat processed food, heavy, oily, fried food, dairy food, nuts, bread, pastries, sugar, red meat, eggs and root vegetables. Have lots of ginger and other warming foods and spices to reduce *Kapha*, unless you have high *Pitta*.
• Drink ginger, cinnamon, cumin, cardamom or fennel tea regularly throughout the day.
• Use warm oil massage (*Abhyanga*) and massage of the energy points on the body (*Marma*) to help

remove blockages and clear *Ama* from the body.

• Take plenty of exercise, such as walking and yoga, and practise *Pranayama* (breathing exercises).

• Scrape your tongue with a tongue-scraper morning and night.

Increasing *Agni* is the key to burning away *Ama*. *Agni* is increased by pungent, sour and salty tastes and by a small amount of bitter taste. Spices are the best thing for increasing *Agni*. They generally have the same qualities as *Agni*, being hot, dry, light and fragrant. With their antimicrobial properties, they help to clear *Ama* and rebalance the gut flora. Turmeric, cinnamon, ginger and long pepper enhance the secretion of digestive enzymes and can be added daily to your food.

Bitter and pungent herbs generally have the ability to clear *Ama* from the gastrointestinal tract. Popular remedies for raising digestive fire and clearing *Ama* include: Trikatu (ginger, long pepper and black pepper); Trikulu (clove, cinnamon and cardamom); pippali; ginger; and Hingwashtaka Churna (asafoetida, ginger, cumin, rock salt, etc.). For more on detoxification, see Chapter 11.

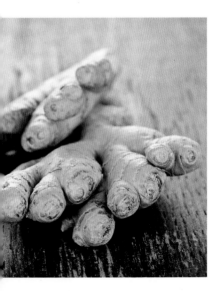

Warming spices, like ginger, not only enkindle Agni *but also clear* Ama.

Chapter 6: Food and your constitution

As the ancient Ayurvedic text, the Sushrita Samhita, stated: 'He whose *doshas* are in balance, whose appetite is good...whose body, mind and senses remain full of bliss, is called a healthy person.'

The six tastes (*Rasa*)

Rasa is the Sanskrit word that means both 'taste' and 'emotion'. This suggests that taste and emotion correspond to one another. An emotion tends to produce in the body its corresponding taste, just as eating foods or herbs of a specific taste tends to create certain emotions.

Ayurveda classifies foods and remedies according to six tastes: sweet, sour, salty, pungent, bitter and astringent. Actually each substance in nature is composed of all five elements, although one or two may predominate. So,

when we experience a food as sour, it means it is mainly sour, but contains other secondary tastes. Certain tastes are better for different people, depending on their basic *Prakruti* (constitution) or their *Vikruti* (*doshic* imbalance).

Understanding the effects on mind and body of each taste, and how this relates to the balance of the *doshas*, means that food and herbs can be specifically related to the needs of each individual, making them more effective tools for the prevention and treatment of imbalance and disease.

The six tastes and the elements

According to Ayurveda, everything in creation is composed of the five

Saffron has pungent, bitter and sweet tastes and is good for all three doshas.

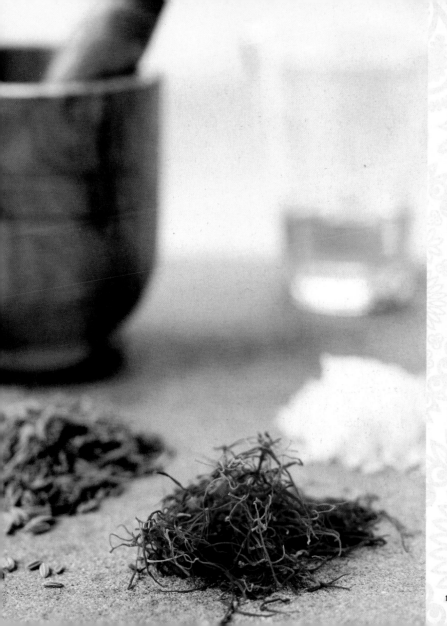

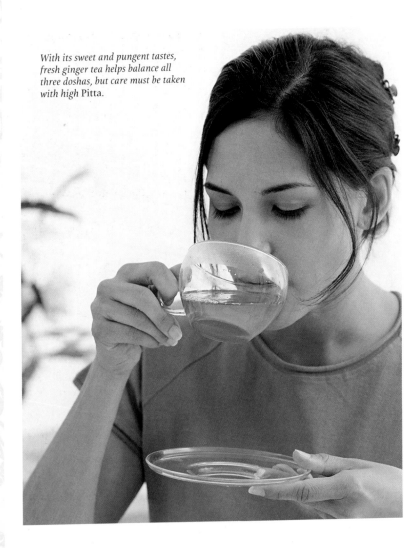

With its sweet and pungent tastes, fresh ginger tea helps balance all three doshas, but care must be taken with high Pitta.

elements found in nature (see page 28) – ether, air, fire, water and earth – and each taste is composed of a combination of two of these elements. The five elements also relate to the three *doshas*, so this means that the amount of each *dosha* that your body produces depends primarily on which tastes you consume.

THE *DOSHAS* AND THE SIX TASTES

- **Sweet, sour and salty tastes** – increase *Kapha* and decrease *Vata*
- **Pungent, bitter and astringent tastes** – decrease *Kapha* and increase *Vata*
- **Sweet, bitter and astringent tastes** – decrease *Pitta*
- **Pungent, sour and salty tastes** – increase *Pitta*

THE ELEMENTS AND THE SIX TASTES

Ether and air / Bitter (*Tikta*)

Air and fire / Pungent (*Katu*)

Fire and water / Salty (*Lavana*)

Water and earth / Sweet (*Madhura*)

Earth and fire / Sour (*Amla*)

Earth and air / Astringent (*Kasaya*)

Sweet

Composed mainly of the elements earth and water, the sweet taste has the effect of increasing *Kapha* and decreasing *Pitta* and *Vata*. Since its qualities (*gunas*) are cooling, heavy and unctuous, it reduces *Agni* (digestive fire).

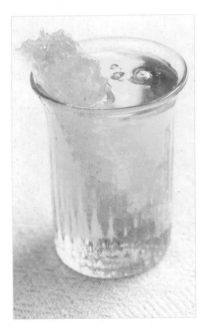

Honey has both sweet and astringent tastes and is actually excellent for Kapha.

Most people love the sweet taste finding it comforting and filling. Naturally sweet-tasting foods (not refined sugar) are nourishing and soothing to body and mind. They relieve hunger and thirst and produce a feeling of satiety in body and mind after digestion. They promote growth, strength and development of all tissues, and increase body weight and fluids so they increase *Kapha*, but are good for *Vata*. Sweet-tasting foods enhance strength and vitality, lubricate skin and hair, nourish the sense organs and make us feel happy.

Overindulgence in sweet food, which is cold, damp and heavy, can lead to lethargy, being overweight,

SWEET-TASTING FOODS

- Most vegetables (particularly root vegetables, such as parsnips, beetroot, sweet potatoes, carrots); pumpkin and butternut squash; sweet fruits such as figs, dates, apricots, pears and prunes; nuts and seeds; oils; grains (especially cooked oats); meat and fish; eggs; milk (except soya); sweeteners (sugar, maple syrup and honey).

- Sweet herbs and spices such as fennel, nutmeg, mint, bala, ashwagandha, shatavari, gokshura, cardamom, vidari, basil, cinnamon.

heaviness, complacency, colds, catarrh and a tendency to constipation. It lowers the digestive fire and can predispose to lymphatic congestion, diabetes, obesity and fibrocystic breast disease. Too many sweet foods increase the complacency of *Kapha*, cool the anger of *Pitta* and comfort the anxiety of *Vata*.

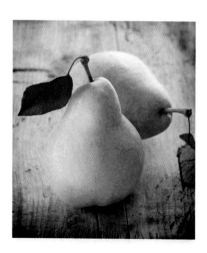

Pears are sweet and astringent and help balance all three doshas.

Sour

Composed mainly of earth and fire, the sour taste increases *Pitta* and *Kapha* and decreases *Vata*. Its qualities (*gunas*) are heating, heavy and unctuous.

Sour-tasting foods and herbs have a refreshing effect, stimulating the mind, enhancing the elimination of wastes and increasing the flow of saliva and other digestive juices. They increase the appetite, improve digestion and absorption and regulate peristalsis. They build up all tissues except the reproductive tissues, increasing energy and vitality and strengthening the heart. They have a grounding effect in *Vata* types.

Sour foods have a warm and damp effect, and in excess they can overheat the digestive tract and cause indigestion, heartburn and acidity. They can also increase the tendency to skin problems, such as acne, boils, urticaria, eczema and psoriasis, aggravate arthritis and cause the teeth to be oversensitive.

After digestion, sour foods are said to increase the desire for more – whether food or general acquisitiveness. Sour causes an evaluation of things in order to determine their desirability. An overindulgence in evaluation is said to lead to envy or jealousy, which may manifest as deprecation of the thing that is desired (as in the 'sour grapes' syndrome). This can increase *Kapha*'s acquisitiveness, if envy of another's success incites us to obtain more for ourselves. *Pitta* can increase if jealousy changes into anger or resentment. It is said that envy may help reduce *Vata* by focusing the mind and motivating consistent action.

SOUR-TASTING FOODS

- **Fermented foods** such as vinegar, wine, cheese, yoghurt, soy sauce, pickles and chutneys; spinach; sour, acidic fruits such as citrus fruits and sour apples, strawberries, green grapes, plums, oranges, raspberries, blueberries and blackberries.

- **Sour herbs and spices** such as amalaki, haritaki, pomegranate.

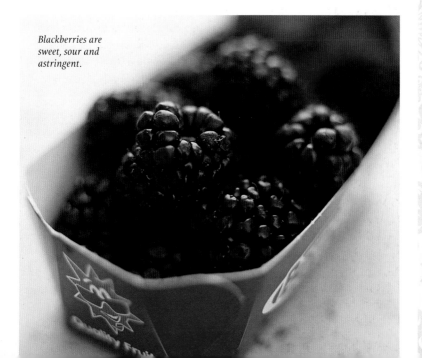

Blackberries are sweet, sour and astringent.

Salty

Composed mainly of water and fire, salty-tasting foods and herbs increase *Kapha* and *Pitta* and decrease *Vata*. Their qualities (*gunas*) are heavy, heating and unctuous.

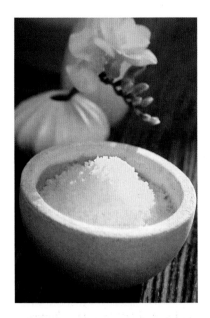

Salt brings out all the flavours of our food, but adding too much to food can have adverse effects.

Salty is called *Sarva Rasa* in Sanskrit, which means 'all tastes', because it can enhance all flavours in food, while at the same time increasing our appetite for food. This is confirmed by our love of salt to enliven crisps and nuts, and by the overuse of salt in the fast-food trade.

Generally it is rock salt or sea salt that is used. In small amounts the salty taste promotes appetite, digestion and absorption, while in large amounts it aggravates *Pitta* symptoms such as acidity, heat, inflammation and rashes. It also aids the elimination of wastes, thereby having a detoxifying effect. Salt has a hydroscopic action, retaining fluids in the

SALTY-TASTING FOODS

• **Salty foods** such as salt, seaweeds; celery; smoked meats and fish; Marmite, yeast extract; anchovies; olives; salted nuts and crisps; cheeses; pickles; fast and processed foods.

• **Salty herbs and spices** such as kelp, celery seed, ajwain seeds, dill seeds, cumin seeds and coriander seeds.

body. This can dilute saliva and phlegm and loosen dense materials that can clog the body.

Too much salt is said to have a depleting effect and to weaken the muscles, and it can cause premature ageing, wrinkles and grey hair. Excess salty foods increase water retention and can predispose us to high blood pressure.

The salty taste is associated with zest for life, which enhances all appetites. It can have a calming and grounding effect, and can reduce the tendency to anxiety, spasms and cramps, which is why it may be helpful for *Vata*.

Due to its heavy, damp and warming properties, those with excess *Pitta* and *Kapha* need to be careful about eating too much salty food. Small amounts of salt can open up blocked channels and increase the mind's desire for intensity of experience. Overindulgence is said to lead to hedonism, which distracts the mind and makes the mind weak.

Too much salt is said to increase complacency and other *Kapha* attributes. It also increases the fieriness of *Pitta*'s anger whenever there is an obstruction to gratification.

Pungent

Composed mainly of fire and air, the pungent taste increases *Pitta* and *Vata*, and decreases *Kapha*. Its qualities (*gunas*) are heating, light and dry.

Pungent foods and herbs stimulate the flow of digestive juices, improving appetite, digestion and absorption. They promote movement, clear channels and obstructions, flush secretions from the body and reduce *Kapha*-like secretions such as mucus, semen, milk and fat. They exert an irritant action on tissues and organs.

Pungent herbs and foods help to destroy bacteria and parasites, and their heating effect causes the eyes to water and the nose to run, and increases circulation and sweating. They stimulate the mind and senses and help to reduce obesity.

On a mental and emotional level, pungency is associated with extroversion, the tendency to excitement and stimulation and particularly with the craving for intensity, too much of which can lead to irritability, impatience and anger and eventually depletion.

Pungent foods, such as chillies, coffee and alcohol, are often loved by those with high *Pitta*, but with their heating effect they are best avoided by them as they can overheat body and mind. Pungency relieves *Kapha* by increasing motivation, and temporarily relieves *Vata* by enhancing self-expression. In the long run it increases *Vata* by overstimulating and dispersing energy. It can increase the tendency in *Vata* types to restlessness, anxiety and insomnia, leaving them depleted and exhausted. Excess pungent foods can cause diarrhoea, heartburn, dry skin, other skin problems and lowered fertility.

PUNGENT-TASTING FOODS

- Pungent foods such as alcohol, raw onions and leeks, mustard greens, radish, watercress, rocket, mustard, horseradish, coffee.

- Pungent herbs and spices include garlic, ginger, basil, black pepper, caraway, cayenne, cinnamon, cloves, cumin, nutmeg, peppermint, saffron, guggulu, fennel, turmeric, chitrak.

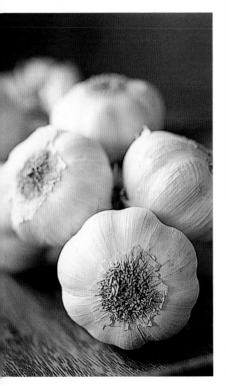

With its strongly pungent taste, garlic stimulates the circulation, decongests the respiratory tract and increases energy and vitality.

Bitter

Composed mainly of air and ether, the bitter taste increases *Vata* and decreases *Pitta* and *Kapha*. Its qualities (*gunas*) are cooling, light and dry.

Bitter is considered the best of all six tastes. Bitter-tasting foods and herbs in small amounts are said to return all tastes to normal and decrease food cravings. Bitter tastes increase the appetite, improve digestion and have a detoxifying effect. Bitter herbs are often used to clear *Ama* (toxins), parasites and other micro-organisms in the gut. The bitter taste also affects the liver, stimulating the flow of bile and supporting the liver in its detoxifying work.

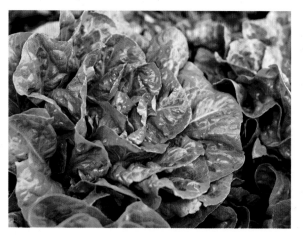

With its bitter taste, lettuce has a detoxifying effect but too much can aggravate Vata.

BITTER-TASTING FOODS

- Bitter food such as coffee, tea; dandelion coffee, aloe-vera juice, chamomile tea; dark chocolate; lettuce, radicchio, chicory, dandelion greens.

- Bitter herbs and spices such as burdock, guduchi, bringaraj, neem, andrographis, coriander, fenugreek, guggulu, bhumiamalaki.

Bitter foods and herbs reduce inflammation and are helpful in the treatment of skin disease and fevers. They reduce fat, sweat and mucus, help to maintain firm skin, reduce weight and aid the elimination of excess water and other elements from the body. Too much bitter, however, can reduce *Agni*, aggravate *Vata* and have a depleting effect on the body and mind.

On a mental and emotional level, the bitter taste is associated with dissatisfaction, which promotes a desire to change. Swallowing a bitter pill means dispelling delusion and facing reality. By stimulating a desire for change, the bitter taste can reduce the complacency of *Kapha*, but overuse increases *Vata*, as dissatisfaction and continuous change can increase insecurity and anxiety.

On a spiritual level, bitter herbs are used in practices in many cultures to increase perception and awareness of how things really are.

Astringent

Composed mainly of air and earth, the astringent taste increases *Vata* and decreases *Pitta and Kapha*. Its qualities (*gunas*) are cooling, light and dry.

Foods and herbs that taste astringent reduce saliva and other secretions and cause a dry, puckering sensation in the mouth. They tone and constrict all parts of the body, reducing secretions such as excess mucus. Their styptic (blood-staunching) properties promote the healing of wounds and reduce bleeding. They help to reduce excess water by their drying effect, so they are recommended for *Kapha*. By their toning effect on the mucous membranes in the gut they protect the gut lining from irritation, inflammation and infection, and heal *Pitta* problems such as gastritis, ulceration, inflammation and diarrhoea. They also help with excessive sweat and saliva. However, excess astringent-tasting foods and herbs inhibit the excretion of faeces, urine and sweat and cause an accumulation of toxins in the body.

On a mental and emotional level, the astringent taste has a cooling and clearing effect, which is good for *Pitta* and *Kapha*, but too much astringency is associated with introversion, shrinking away from excitement and stimulation. Astringency is not good for *Vata*. Too much introversion can increase the insecurity, anxiety and fear that characterizes *Vata* types, and is associated with neuromuscular disorders.

Pomegranates have an astringent taste and are packed with antioxidants.

ASTRINGENT-TASTING FOODS

- **Astringent food** such as dry red wine; unripe bananas; beans and pulses; honey; apples and pears; foods from the cabbage family – cabbage, broccoli, Brussels sprouts and cauliflower; sloes, pomegranates, cranberries; alfalfa sprouts, green beans, peas; Jerusalem artichokes; potatoes; buckwheat.

- **Astringent herbs and spices** such as haritaki, rose, musta, jasmine, ashoka, guggulu, bibhitaki.

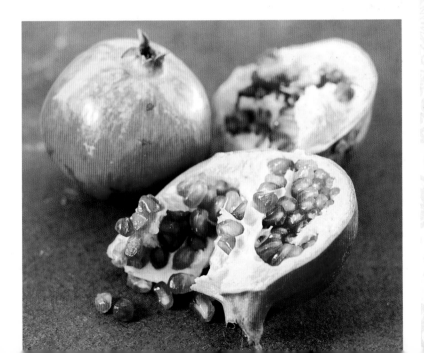

The effects of food and herbs

When taste is experienced in the mouth it is transmitted to the brain, which determines the type of substances that have been ingested and the digestive enzymes needed for optimal digestion. By the time the food reaches the gut, the digestive organs should be prepared. So it is important that you taste properly the food you are eating.

According to Ayurveda there are three different effects of food and herbs:

1 *Rasa*, or taste – the effect that foods and herbs have before digestion, determined by the taste buds while food is in the mouth.

2 *Virya*, or energy – experienced during digestion. Hot food increases the body's ability to digest, freeing energy for other metabolic tasks. Cold food requires extra energy for its digestion, obtained from the rest of the body, which must reduce its other activities as a result.

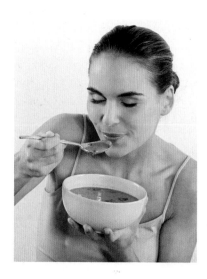

Hot food, like soup, is much easier to digest than cold food.

3 *Vipaka*, or post-digestive effect – when the nutrients are assimilated after digestion, deep within the tissues.

Balancing effects

A substance may have a heating taste and cold energy, meaning that initially it increases digestion but does not aggravate *Pitta*. It may have a cooling taste and hot energy, like the bitter taste, reducing the appetite, but increasing digestion.

Cooling tastes (sweet, bitter and astringent) have a cold and contracting effect on the emotions, decreasing our desire to eat more. Heating tastes have a hot and expansive effect, increasing our desire to eat more.

Salty is the taste to balance *Vata*, as it is heavy, oily, heating and improves digestion; sour comes next, then sweet. Bitter is the best taste to balance *Pitta*; then sweet, then astringent. Pungent is the best taste to balance *Kapha*; bitter comes next, then astringent.

THE THREE EFFECTS

Taste	Energy	Post-digestive effect
Sweet	Cooling	Sweet
Sour	Hot	Sour
Salty	Hot	Sweet
Pungent	Hot	Pungent
Bitter	Cooling	Pungent
Astringent	Cooling	Pungent

People with a *Pitta* constitution should drink water after meals to prevent acid indigestion and disorders such as eye diseases, headaches and piles; consuming hot food and drinks in excess increases *Pitta*.

Taking excessive cold food and drinks gives rise to *Kapha* and *Vata* diseases, such as anorexia, colicky pain, hiccups, headaches, lethargy and disturbed bowels.

Chapter 7: **Preventative health**

Our daily activities clearly have an effect on our general health. In Ayurveda there are distinct guidelines for a healthy lifestyle that address almost every aspect of daily living, and these form the basis of preventative medicine.

Our *Dinacharya*, or daily routine, is intended to keep the three *doshas* in a state of healthy equilibrium, and our digestion and metabolism (*Agni*) balanced. In Sanskrit, *din* means 'day' and *acharya* means 'behaviour' or 'to follow'.

If you adopt a daily routine you can structure your life to fit in all the things you want to do, as well as those you need to do to keep yourself happy and healthy. You can plan at what time it feels best to get up and when it suits you to go to bed. It may be helpful to make a list of all that you would like to have in your life at the moment, on a daily or weekly basis, and then make sure that you give these things a place in your routine. You could then call *Dinacharya* 'doing what you dream'!

Getting up between 6 and 7 a.m. and going to bed by 10 p.m. is the ideal Ayurvedic way.

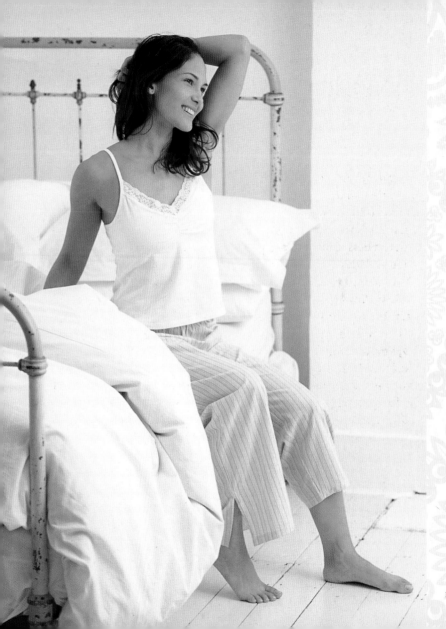

Ayurvedic daily routine (*Dinacharya*)

Dinacharya takes into the account the relationship between the *doshas* and the time of day. Each day we experience six different phases, which relate to the preponderance of the *doshas* at that time.

At dawn, when the sun is about to rise, the dry, cold, mobile aspects of *Vata* that have accumulated through the night are prevalent. *Vata* predominates between 2 and 6 a.m. In the early morning the cool and heavy energy of *Kapha* can make us feel sluggish, if we stay in bed too long into *Kapha* time (6–10 a.m.). At midday, when the sun is at its peak, *Pitta* predominates. In the early afternoon the energy of *Vata* once more dominates. In the evening, when the heaviness of *Kapha* returns, it induces a feeling of relaxation and is a good time to rest. At midnight, when the sun is furthest away from the earth, *Pitta* predominates again.

Your routine

Structure and routine are very good for those with a predominantly *Vata* constitution as they help them to remain calm and focused. They enable *Pitta* types to cope better with the many things they want

---

THE *DOSHAS* AND THEIR TIMES OF DAY

Vata: Dominant 2 a.m.–6 a.m. and 2 p.m.–6 p.m.

Pitta: Dominant 10 a.m.–2 p.m. and 10 p.m.–2 a.m.

Kapha: Dominant 6 a.m.–10 a.m. and 6 p.m.–10 p.m.

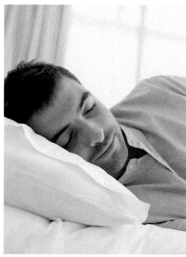

It is best to go to sleep as near to 10 p.m. as possible before Pitta *energy gives you a second wind.*

Guidelines for healthy living

Below are the Ayurvedic guidelines for healthy living, which can help you to formulate your own *Dinarcharya* that suits you and your present life. Starting and ending the day with prayer, meditation, *Pranayama* (breathing exercises) or a ritual of your own choosing helps to balance your spiritual and material life.

Arising

To attune your biological clock to those of nature and the sun, it is generally best to wake just before sunrise or between 6 and 7 a.m.

Natural urges

The early hours of the morning from 2 a.m. to 6 a.m. are ruled by *Vata*, which governs elimination;

to cram in and to feel a sense of accomplishment at the end of the day. For those who are predominantly *Kapha*, a daily routine helps to energize and motivate them. Generally speaking, it is best to do work that involves mental focus and concentration in the morning, physical things in the afternoon and then in the evening, after a day's work and after eating, to relax so that you can wind down before sleep.

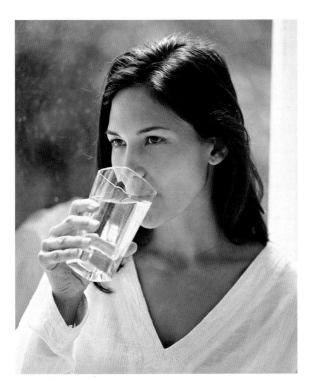

Drinking a glass of lukewarm water first thing in the morning helps to flush out toxins.

so the best time to empty the bowels is on rising, early in the morning, and this also helps clear *Kapha* that has accumulated during sleep, helping you to feel awake and alert. Then wash your face and hands with cool water, rosewater or a decoction of amalaki. Never suppress natural physical urges, such as emptying the bowels, passing water, eating when hungry, drinking when thirsty, sleeping when tired, sneezing, yawning, burping, crying or passing wind, as it aggravates *Vata* and so adversely affects the other *doshas*.

Drinking water

Drinking a glass of lukewarm water helps to flush out toxins accumulated overnight. Those with a *Pitta* constitution should take cool water first thing in the morning. For all constitutions, when taken in through the nose using a *Neti* pot (a little metal pot like an Aladdin's lamp), water is said to improve the eyesight and is good for the sinuses. It helps to prevent congestion and respiratory infections.

Teeth

According to Ayurveda, teeth are a by-product of bone. Neem and liquorice stems can be chewed and used as a toothbrush. A toothpaste can be made from sesame oil mixed with fine powder of ginger, black pepper, long pepper, cardamom, Triphala and rock salt. Ground almond shell is also used to make tooth powder in India.

Cavities in the teeth and receding gums are signs of *Vata* aggravation in the skeletal system, and are often related to a deficiency of calcium, magnesium and zinc. To prevent these problems, chew a handful of calcium-rich black sesame seeds every morning, then brush your teeth without toothpaste so that the residue of the sesame seeds is rubbed against the teeth, polishing and cleaning them.

To prevent receding gums, tooth infection and cavities, you can massage the gums daily with sesame oil or with Triphala powder mixed with sesame oil. Sesame oil nourishes bone tissue (*Asthi dhatu*). Take a mouthful of sesame oil and swish it from side to side for two or three minutes, then spit out the oil. Then gently massage the gums with the index finger. Chewing food well stimulates the gums and helps to keep them healthy. Eating four figs every day is said to strengthen teeth and gums alike.

Eyes

Anu-taila oil (a combination of many different herbs) in the nose and sesame oil in the ears is said to be good for the eyes; and a quarter to half a teaspoon of Triphala taken regularly at night with honey and ghee is a good eye tonic. Milk with shatavari is also recommended for the eyes. Adequate sleep is important. Looking at or touching auspicious objects is also said to be good for the mind.

Oiling the head

Applying oil that is applicable to your constitution on your head helps to maintain healthy hair and scalp and prevent headaches, hair loss and greying. When applied before bed, it also helps sleep.

Ears

Sesame or coconut oil can be dropped into the ears daily. It is particularly good for reducing *Vata* symptoms such as hearing problems, tinnitus and wax accumulation.

Nose

Two drops of anu-taila oil in each nostril each morning after bathing or before going to bed are

Daily self-massage of the body with sesame oil has a rejuvenating and health-promoting effect.

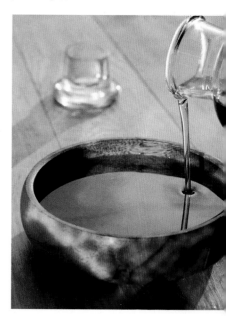

Gargling with sesame oil helps fight off the viruses and bacteria that are responsible for colds and throat infections.

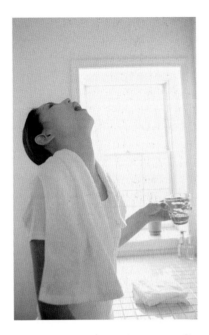

recommended. Using nose drops is known as *Nasya* and it is especially good for reducing *Vata* disturbances of the mind and head, as well as preventing respiratory infections. Those with a *Pitta* constitution or a tendency to nosebleeds can use ghee mixed with a little saffron. For a dry nose that tends to block easily, sesame oil medicated with bala can be used as nose drops. *Bhastrika* – forceful expiration from each nostril with the mouth closed – keeps the air passages clean and helps to prevent respiratory infections (for more on *Pranayama* see page 278).

Voice

Sucking cloves is recommended for the voice. Two drops of anu-taila oil in the throat, and gargling with sesame oil medicated with clove or rose, is also recommended. Avoid cold drinks and ice cream.

Gargling

After brushing your teeth, you can rinse the mouth, scrape the tongue and gargle with water. Sesame oil is particularly recommended for warding off infection.

Oil massage

Self-massage of the body with sesame oil for 15 minutes every day before a bath or shower improves the skin, tones the muscles and blood vessels and has a soothing action on the nervous system. If you are short of time, simply drop a little sesame oil in the ears and massage the neck, head, spine and soles.

Sesame-oil massage just three times a week will have a beneficial effect. It is particularly calming for *Vata*. It stimulates the circulation, helps the removal of wastes from the tissues, improves vision, enhances the five senses, induces restful sleep and helps to delay ageing. Oil massage of the soles relieves lethargy and fatigue, and is good for the nerves and eyes. It can be done in all seasons except hot summer.

Exercise

Exercise should be taken regularly in the morning until you perspire or mouth-breathe. Vigorous exercise is best taken in winter and spring. Regular exercise increases stamina and resistance to disease by enhancing immunity, clearing the channels, and promoting the circulation and elimination of wastes. It can also reduce the tendency to depression and anxiety. Depending on age, *Kapha* people can take more heavy exercise; *Pitta* types should take moderate, uncompetitive exercise; and *Vata* types should do gentle walking or yoga.

Yoga is good for the spine and organs of digestion, respiration and so on, and helps to calm the mind. Sun salutations get your *Prana* (energy) moving, remove stagnation in your body and strengthen your digestive fire.

Avoid any kind of exercise if you are unwell, and immediately after a meal. *Pranayama* wakes you up, clears the mind and oxygenates the body, helping to enhance physical and mental stamina.

Bathing

A bath is recommended after oil massage, using warm water for your body and cool water for your head. You can use a scrub for the skin made from a paste of devadaru, and amalaki.

Warm water medicated with holy basil leaves is good for a *Vata* constitution. Those with a *Pitta* constitution can use cool water with sandalwood or manjishta. *Kapha* people are best with hot water medicated with kadambari (*Anthocephalus indicus*) or pepper.

Bathing purifies the senses, dispels fatigue and increases *Ojas* (strength, the body's prime energy reserve). After your bath is the best time for meditation or prayer.

A warm, relaxing bath after oil massage nourishes Ojas.

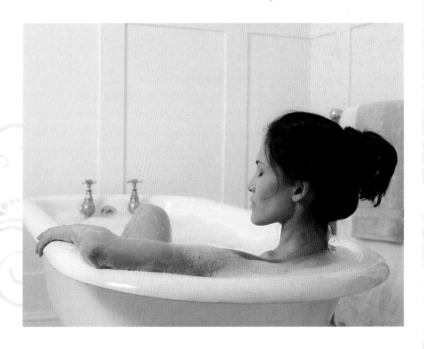

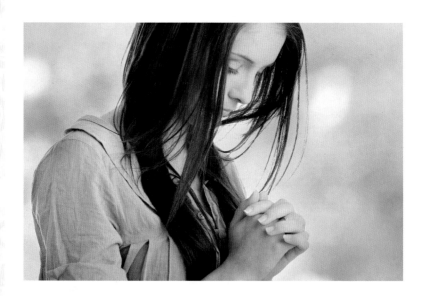

Clothing

Ideally clothing should be light, unless the weather is very cold, and made of natural fibres such as cotton, wool, linen or silk. The skin needs to breathe and allow the blood to circulate freely.

Diet

We need to eat regularly, leaving four to six hours between meals and at least three hours between the last meal and going to bed. As well as modifying your diet according to your *doshic* constitution, you should vary it according to your state of health and the season.

It is important to eat slowly, chewing each mouthful so that you can digest and absorb your food. Eat quietly, without doing anything else at the same time, such as reading or watching

154

The best time for meditation or prayer is after bathing.

television, and taste and enjoy your food. Heavy foods are best avoided at night. After lunch you can take a short walk to stimulate the digestion. In the evening you can stroll in the fresh air to refresh mind and body. Before bed you can pray or meditate again.

Meditation or prayer

After bathing, sit in a comfortable position with your spine straight. Calm your mind and focus on your breath or your mantra. This is ideal for disciplining the mind, increasing awareness and clarity and reducing stress.

Sleep

A calm mind, oil massage, instilling oil drops in the ear, a bath, a good dinner and a comfortable bed in a soothing environment should help ensure a good night's sleep. It is best to go to sleep at the same time each night, if possible, preferably by 10 p.m. before going into *Pitta* time and to ensure eight hours of sleep. Taking half a teaspoon of ashwagandha in warm milk before bed will help ensure a restful sleep. Brahmi, nutmeg and shankapushpi are also helpful.

Rejuvenatives

Tonic herbs that are renowned for their ability to improve the quality of the tissues can be taken regularly. They include ashwagandha, bibhitaki, pippali, shatavari, gotu kola, amalaki, haritaki, liquorice, guduchi, bala, gokshura, punarnava and the formula Chayawanprash. *Rasayanas*, or rejuvenative tonics, can be physical as well as more subtle.

Spending time outside in nature, as well as love, compassion, caring for others, studying and aspiring to self-knowledge and the practice of meditation, also act as *Rasayanas* (see page 370).

Seasonal variations (*Parinam*)

The three *doshas* are affected by a season's heat/cold, wet/dry and heavy/light qualities. At certain times the *doshas* accumulate, at others they are aggravated and at other times they are alleviated.

SEASONAL EFFECTS

Late winter/ spring	*Pitta* accumulates, *Kapha* aggravated, *Vata* calm
Summer	*Pitta* aggravated, Vata accumulates, *Kapha* calm
Autumn	*Vata* aggravated, *Pitta* and *Kapha* calm
Winter	*Kapha* accumulates, *Vata* and *Pitta* calm

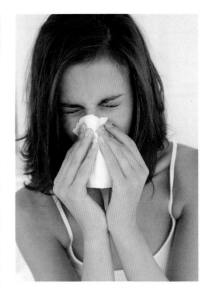

Illness is much more likely to occur at the junctions of seasons, when Vata is aggravated.

Foods eaten and herbs taken in a particular season are best chosen according to their qualities. Substances selected should have the qualities opposite to the season. If the weather is cold and damp, foods and herbs that are warm, dry and reduce *Kapha* are indicated. If diet, lifestyle and routine are not adjusted according to the season to maintain the equilibrium of the *doshas*, it may adversely affect your health.

Seasonal routines need to account for constitutional differences. A healthy person should adjust their food and lifestyle to balance *Kapha* in late winter and spring, *Pitta* during the summer and *Vata* during autumn and early winter, while a strongly *Vata*, *Pitta* or *Kapha* person needs to balance their predominant *dosha* all year round.

Illness is more likely to occur at the junctions of the seasons, which are times of *Vata* aggravation. Ovulation and menstruation are junctions of the menstrual cycle; dawn and dusk are junctions of the day and night; adolescence and menopause are the junctions of life. Seasonal detoxification helps to protect against illness developing at such times (see page 204).

At the junction of winter and spring *Kapha* becomes predominant, and this is the best time for all constitutions to clear *Kapha*. Someone with a *Kapha* constitution requires more strenuous purification than a *Pitta* person, who is best purified with mild purgation. It is best for a *Vata* person to gradually eliminate *Kapha* with gentle medicines and a *Kichari* fast (see page 215) than use stronger measures, which may increase *Vata*. Between spring and summer both *Pitta* and *Kapha* types may profit from purgation, which may or may not be suitable for a *Vata* person, according to their specific condition. *Vata* people respond well to medicated enemas at the junction between autumn and winter.

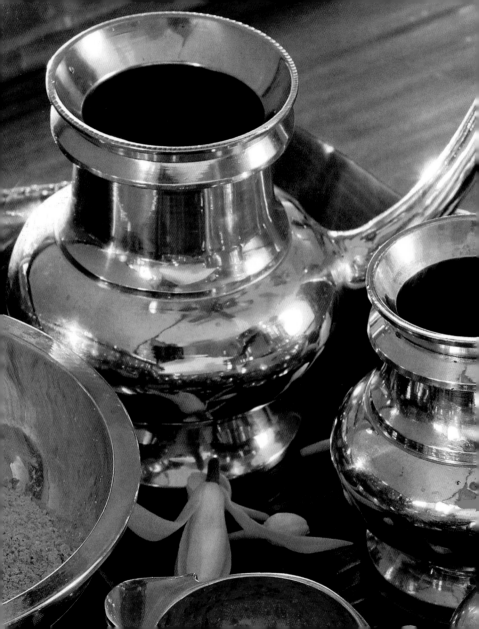

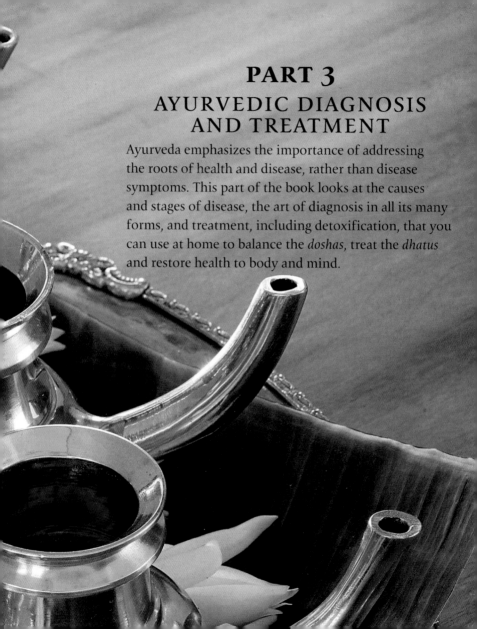

PART 3
AYURVEDIC DIAGNOSIS AND TREATMENT

Ayurveda emphasizes the importance of addressing the roots of health and disease, rather than disease symptoms. This part of the book looks at the causes and stages of disease, the art of diagnosis in all its many forms, and treatment, including detoxification, that you can use at home to balance the *doshas*, treat the *dhatus* and restore health to body and mind.

Chapter 8: **The causes and stages of disease (*Samprapti*)**

According to Ayurveda, the cause of disease (*Vyadhi*) is the impaired equilibrium of the three *doshas*, which then disturbs the digestive fire (*Agni*) and leads to the formation of toxins (*Ama*), which affects the nourishment and health of the tissues (*dhatus*). The imbalance of *doshas* and the course they follow to cause disease is termed *Samprapti*, or pathogenesis.

Unique to Ayurveda is the understanding that all diseases pass through the same six stages and, at each of the first five levels, the disease can be halted and addressed, if the right changes in diet and lifestyle are made. Herbs can also be used to balance the *doshas* and *Agni*, clear *Ama* and nourish the *dhatus*, bringing body and mind back into balance.

There is a range of different herbs that can be made into teas to balance the constitution.

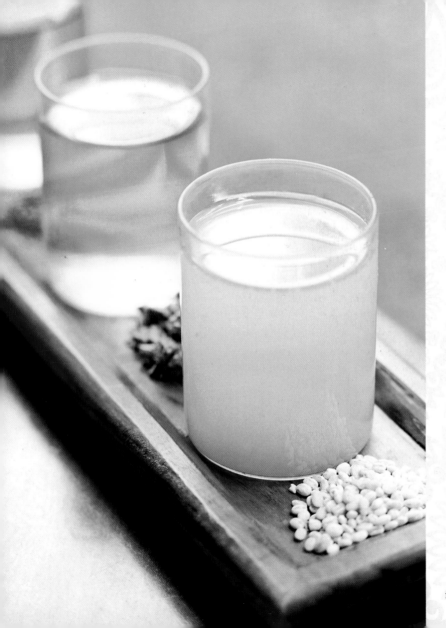

The six stages of disease

The benefit of recognizing the stages that disease goes through as it develops is that early signs of ill health can be detected before they become hard to treat or so fixed in the body that they are untreatable. It enables the correct preventative and curative measures to be taken.

Ascertaining the stage of any disease gives a clear indication of the prognosis – meaning how quickly and effectively you will recover from the symptoms you are experiencing.

The three early stages of disease are represented by vague and ill-defined symptoms, which often lie below the threshold of awareness. Only the three last stages give rise to clear symptoms that are normally associated with illness. If subtle imbalances can be perceived in the first three stages, then you can take steps to remedy the situation and prevent full-blown disease.

According to Ayurveda, all disturbances of the *doshas* start with the mind and specifically with:

• *Avidhya:* Ignorance – we take in the wrong information about what is right for our health and act accordingly.

• *Asatya indrya samartha:* Misappropriate attachment of the senses – we make incorrect judgments, such as drinking excess alcohol, thinking it is a good thing, even though it is harmful and addictive.

• *Prajna paradha:* 'Crimes against wisdom' – we don't learn from experience and repeat the same mistakes, such as drinking alcohol and suffering from a hangover, or eating sugar even though last time it gave us a hyperglycaemic attack.

Such 'crimes against wisdom' lead to the six stages of disease, as follows:

1 Accumulation (*Chaya*)
2 Aggravation (*Prakopa*)
3 Overflow (*Prasara*)
4 Relocation (*Sthansan shraya*)
5 Manifestation (*Vyakti*)
6 Diversification/specification (*Bheda*).

Accumulation: The first stage involves an increase, accumulation and stagnation of the *dosha* in its main site in the body:

• The lower abdomen for *Vata*
• The mid-abdomen, stomach, small intestine, liver and so on for *Pitta*

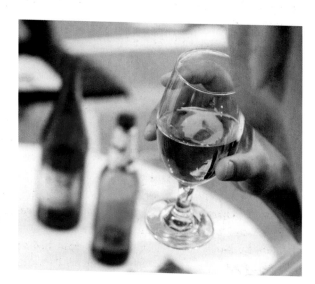

We can make errors of judgment, thinking that drinking alcohol is good for us.

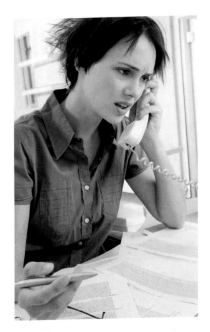

Stress can further provoke the dosha *imbalance and lead to aggravation and overflow.*

give rise to bloating, wind or constipation; increased *Pitta* may involve an increased feeling of heat and a slightly acid stomach; if *Kapha* is raised there might be lethargy, sluggish digestion and catarrh.

Aggravation: The *dosha* becomes further excited. This is provoked by our lifestyle, by stress and specifically by:
• Food (*Ahara*)
• Activity (*Vihara*)
• Seasonal or climatic changes (*Charya*) (see page 204), leading to the following stage of disease.

Overflow: As the *dosha* accumulates further, it overflows from its main site and is distributed to other tissues, particularly if they have an affinity to the *dosha* involved. If *Vata* accumulates, it can overflow from the lower abdomen into the mind, causing anxiety or insomnia, or into the joints, causing aching joints. If *Pitta* overflows from the stomach/small

• The upper stomach and respiratory system for *Kapha*.

No clear signs or symptoms occur at this stage, just an awareness of the increased *dosha*. For example, increased *Vata* may

intestine, it can manifest in irritability and perfectionism, or in skin problems. And if *Kapha* is aggravated, then *Kledaka Kapha* (a subtype of *Kapha* governing digestion) in the stomach can be affected, causing sluggish digestion, lack of appetite and lethargy.

There may be one, two or even three *doshas* involved at the same time, and for many people this can be confusing when it comes to determining which *dosha* to treat first. If the aggravated *dosha* is *Vata*, but has spread over into specific sites of *Pitta* (such as the skin), then the line of treatment should be as for *Pitta*. If the aggravated *dosha* is *Pitta* and has spread over to specific sites of *Kapha* (and vice versa), then it should be treated as for the *dosha* of that site (see subtypes of the *doshas* on page 54).

Relocation: This represents the prodromal (early symptomatic) stage of disease that is yet to manifest as frank symptoms. The excited *dosha*, having overflowed and spread to other parts of the body, becomes localized and marks the beginnings of disease relating to those tissues. It interacts with the *dhatus* (see page 64) in these parts. The sites chosen for the location of the excited *dosha* depend on the strength or weakness of the *dhatus*, and this varies from one person to another. At this stage it is still possible to reverse the process with diet and lifestyle changes and the use of herbs.

Manifestation: The disease is fully manifested by physical symptoms, which occur where the *dosha* has settled, such as in the joints in arthritis or the head in migraine.

Diversification/specification: This is the stage at which the disease may become sub-acute, chronic or incurable. Diet and lifestyle advice and herbs can be used to improve and ease symptoms, but they may never disappear completely.

The pathways of disease

There are three pathways of disease classified in Ayurveda: the inner path (*Antar marga*), the outer path (*Bahya marga*) and the middle path (*Madhyam marga*).

The inner path consists of the digestive tract, which stretches from mouth to anus. It is here that the three *doshas* first accumulate and are disturbed, and it is the site of the first and second stages of disease, accumulation (*Chaya*) and aggravation (*Prakopa*). By using herbs such as Triphala to regulate *Agni* and clear *Ama*, and by adjusting your diet and lifestyle to balance the *doshas*, the excess *doshas* can be effectively cleared from the site and illness averted.

The outer path is the peripheral part of the body and involves the skin, *Rasa* (plasma) and *Rakta* (blood) *dhatus*. Once symptoms appear on the skin, it means that disease has developed into the third stage of disease, overflow (*Prasara*).

Warm-oil massage and steam and fomentation, as well as herbs such as Triphala, can help to move *Ama* back to the inner path, to be eliminated via the bowels.

The middle path involves the vital organs, such as the brain, heart, lungs, liver, kidneys and reproductive organs. It also affects the other *dhatus*: *Mamsa* (muscle tissue), *Medas* (fat tissue), *Asthi* (bone tissue), *Majja* (nervous tissue) and *Shukra* (reproductive tissue). Once the disturbed *dosha(s)* and *Ama* affect the middle path, it means that disease has developed into the fourth and fifth stages, relocation (*Sthansan shraya*) and manifestation (*Vyakti*) and, if left untreated, it can progress to the sixth stage, diversification (*Bheda*).

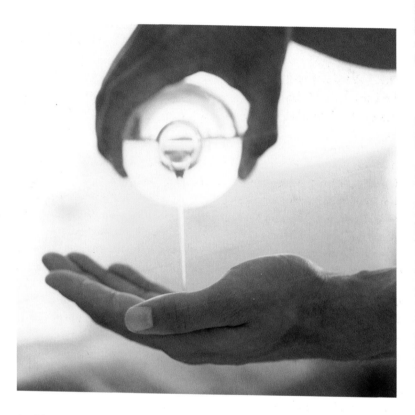

At this stage chronic disease has set in and self-treatment is probably not the best option. You are advised to consult an Ayurvedic practitioner or visit a *Panchakarma* clinic.

Warm-oil massage can help to move Ama back to the inner path to be eliminated.

Chapter 9: **Ayurvedic diagnostic techniques**

Before treatment can begin you need to ascertain your basic constitution (*Prakruti*) and the present imbalance of your *doshas* (*Vikruti*) (see page 96), which may have caused the symptoms or disease (*Roga*) that needs resolving.

It is best to assess your constitution with preventative health in mind, rather than waiting until you actually feel unwell. Good diagnosis is important so that the right preventative and curative measures can be taken, meaning that treatment can be as effective as possible.

Throughout the ancient Ayurvedic texts, such as those by Charaka and Sushrita (see page 15) there is a wealth of information concerning diagnostic techniques, and these are blended by Ayurvedic practitioners with the ever-changing diagnostic measures, as the tradition of Ayurveda keeps pace with modern developments and increased knowledge about the diagnosis of disease. This means that diagnostic methods may vary from one practitioner to another, but broadly they follow the same general lines.

Good diagnosis is important so that the right measures can be taken to correct your individual imbalances.

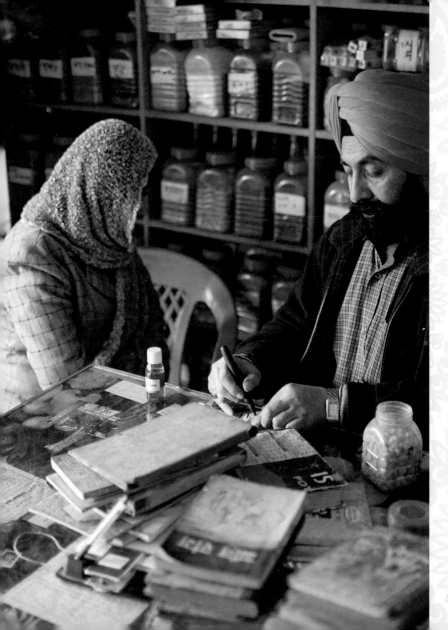

The art of diagnosis

When taking a case history an Ayurvedic practitioner will ask many questions and will also use observation, touch, therapies and 'advising' (prescribing some form of treatment using diet and herbs to balance one or other *dosha* in order to discover what is wrong). If symptoms improve, the practitioner will advise on further treatments along the same lines; if not, they will modify their suggestions.

Through questioning, the practitioner will ascertain the state of the patient's digestion, diet, lifestyle, habits and general strength or resilience. This will give them an idea of the prognosis: how long it will take the patient to recover full health. The physical examination often includes inspecting the patient's urine, stools, tongue, bodily sounds, eyes, skin and general appearance.

Traditionally the art of diagnosis in Ayurveda is divided into two parts: *Rogi pariksa* (the inspection of the person); and *Roga pariksa* (examination of the disease). The Madhava Nidana treatise described five different aspect of diagnosis that are necessary to assess the symptoms, the nature of a person's disease (*Roga*) as well as the root causes, so that treatment can be more effective.

1 Causes of *Roga* (*Nidana* or *Hetu*)

The cause of disease (*Vyadi*) is assessed in terms of the nature of the imbalance of the three *doshas*, which then disturbs the digestive fire (*Agni*) and leads to the formation of toxins (*Ama*), which in turn affects the nourishment and health of the *dhatus* (tissues).

It is vital to establish why you have become unwell so that the underlying causes can be addressed, using the right diet, herbs and lifestyle advice, and to avoid treating solely the symptoms. If the causes are not understood, treatment is unlikely to be effective or a recurrence of the symptoms is probable.

2 Prodromal symptoms (*Purva-Rupa*)

Ayurveda divides the progress of imbalance into full-blown illness through the six stages of disease (see page 162). The first three stages are the prodromal (early symptomatic) stages, which involve vague and ill-defined symptoms that often lie below the threshold of awareness.

An Ayurvedic consultation includes the taking of a full case history using questions and close observation.

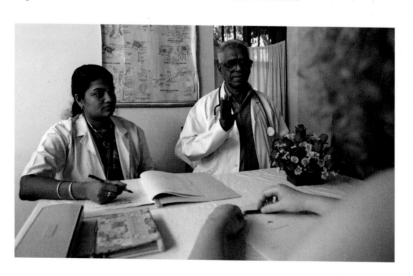

If subtle imbalances that provide useful warnings can be perceived in the first three stages, you can take steps to remedy the situation and full-blown disease can be prevented.

3 Actual signs and symptoms of *Roga* (*Rupa*)

These represent the three last stages of disease and give rise to clear symptoms that are normally associated with illness.

4 Pathogenesis, or the course of disease (*Samprapti*)

The analysis of imbalance of the *doshas*, and the course they have followed to cause disease, is termed *Samprapti* or pathogenesis (see page 160).

5 Therapeutic test (*Upasaya*)

This is the use of exploratory therapy in the form of diet, herbs and lifestyle changes, when the exact diagnosis is unclear, to see whether they help or exacerbate. For example, insomnia that responds to taking ashwagandha in warm milk before bed, or painful joints that are eased by warm-oil massage, indicates clearly that they are caused by an imbalance of *Vata* (air-humour).

Diagnostic tools

According to the major classical text Charaka, three things are essential for diagnosis:

• **Direct observation** (*Pratyaksha*) using the practitioner's five senses – listening, feeling, looking, smelling and tasting. However, in place of the last one modern practitioners use questioning! Practitioners may use stethoscopes and, for the ears, auriculoscopes and magnifying instruments such as otoscopes.

• **Textual authority** (*Shabdha* or *Aptopadesh*), which is twofold. First there is the body of recorded knowledge in the literature of Ayurveda, and the teachings of

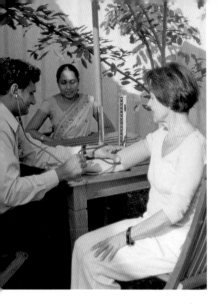

Ayurvedic diagnosis includes a blend of old and new, both traditional and modern practices.

The eightfold examinations

Direct observation consists of 'the eightfold examinations', as follows:

1 Pulse (*Nadi pariksha*): This is a highly developed practical method for increasing insight into the physiology and pathology of the body and mind. It takes years of practice to perfect and includes determining the rate, depth, strength, position and quality of the radial pulse on each wrist, with a view to determining the *Prakruti* and *Vikruti* of the patient, the state of the seven *dhatus*, the strength and resilience of the person.

2 Tongue (*Jibha pariksha*): This includes the shape, colour, coating and specific characteristics, such as tooth marks, lines, cracks, swellings, swellings and raised papillae. It can tell us much about the digestion, the *doshas*, the quality of blood

well-known Ayurvedic physicians. Second there is the information taken by the practitioner during a case history, including past medical and family history.

• **Inference** (*Anumana*) – this means reasoning based on inference, an analysis of all the information gathered through the practitioner's former knowledge and expertise, and through the interview with the patient, including pulse diagnosis. The end result is the diagnosis, prognosis and a plan of treatment.

(*Rakta dhatu*) and whether there is *Ama* (toxins).

3 Urine (*Mutra pariksha*): This includes the colour, odour, volume, frequency and consistency, telling us more about the *doshas*. A unique method of analysis is used to assess the state of the *doshas*. A few drops of oil are added to the urine, when placed in a bowl, and the activity of the oil denotes the *doshic* balance.

4 Faeces (*Mala pariksha*): This includes the regularity, odour, colour, form, consistency and whether or not the stool sinks or floats, which gives information about the digestion and the *doshas*.

5 Body symmetry (*Akruti pariksha*): This includes an assessment of the body's physical proportions, the prominence of bones and veins and the amount of fat, as a further guide to the balance of the *doshas*.

6 Eyes (*Druck pariksha*): This includes the colour, shape, brightness and clarity of the eyes, telling us particularly about the quality of the nervous tissue (*Majja dhatu*). *Vata* signs include dryness and possible tics or twitches; *Pitta* (fire-humour) is indicated by redness and irritation, and *Kapha* (water-humour) by large, but watery, eyes.

7 Voice or sounds (*Shabdha pariksha*): This includes the sound, pitch and volume of the voice, as well as other sounds of the body, such as breathing, intestinal movements and joints, which tell us more about the balance of the *doshas*.

8 Skin (*Sparsha pariksha*): This includes the temperature, texture, dryness, moisture, firmness and smoothness of the skin, telling us about quality of plasma tissue (*Rasa dhatu*).

For a really complete diagnosis the practitioner will also use the Ten Assessments (*Dashavidhya pariksha*).

THE TEN ASSESSMENTS

1 Assessment of the constitution (*Prakruti*): analysis of our basic constitution, *Vata*, *Pitta* or *Kapha*, and combinations of these

2 State of imbalance (*Vikruti*): the present state of imbalances of the *doshas*

3 Quality of the tissues (*Sara*): deficient, excessive and impaired states of the seven *dhatus*

4 Quality of the body (*Sharira sanhana*): the type of build, strength, nutritional status, movement and general functioning

5 Body type (*Sharira pranama*): whether tall, short, stout or thin, in proportion or symmetrical

6 Lifestyle (*Satmya*): daily and seasonal routines, diet, climate, behaviour, likes and dislikes

7 Psychological constitution (*Manas prakruti*): the state of mind and emotions, including the ability to intellectually analyse (*Dee*), memory retention (*Druthi*) and memory recall (*Smriti*). It includes an evaluation of the *gunas* (qualities): *Sattva* (clarity and harmony), *Rajas* (energy and action) and *Tamas* (decay and inertia)

8 Digestive fire (*Sama Agni*): erratic, strong, weak/slow or balanced

9 Energy levels (*Viyayam shakti*): the capacity to exercise, strength and endurance

10 Age (*Vyas*): young, middle-aged or elderly; this can be used to compare your current level of health

Pulse diagnosis (*Nadi pariksha*)

The pulse represents the rhythmical flow of blood as it is pumped from the heart into the arterial system of the body. Its rate and rhythm tell us about the health of the heart and reveal much about the patient's state of mind, since the heart is not merely a pump, but represents the seat of the consciousness.

There are many different methods of pulse-taking, and the pulse varies considerably from one part of the day to the next, so the traditional viewpoint is that pulse diagnosis is an 'inferential' (*Anumana*) method of obtaining knowledge and needs to be considered alongside other methods of diagnosis. As stated in the Ayurveda Saukhyam, 'The examination of the pulse should be conducted with great care. Proficiency is attained only by constant practice'.

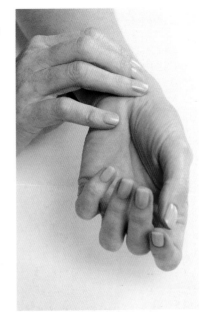

Place the tips of your index, middle and ring fingers over your pulse.

Time

The ideal time to take the pulse is first thing in the morning after emptying your bowels. It is not advisable to take it when you have just done exercise, eaten, drunk something hot, had a hot bath or shower or are feeling stressed, as these make it hard to rely solely on the readings of the pulse.

Position

When taking the pulse, gently place the tips of your index, middle and ring fingers on the surface of the skin over the radial artery in the wrist, and apply pressure evenly in all three places simultaneously. Place your index finger in the distal position (furthest away from the heart) just below the wrist bone, keeping small gaps between the fingers.

You can take one wrist pulse at a time or, ideally (when taking the pulse of someone else), take both wrists at the same time. The pulse on the left side is more indicative of the constitution in women, and that on the right side in men.

Gait (*Gati*)

The gait of the pulse has traditionally been likened to that of different animals:

• A *Vata* **pulse** is said to be like the movement of a snake: thin, weak, thready, wriggling, slipping away under pressure, making it hard to detect. It may be fast and/or irregular, and the patient's skin may be cold and dry to the touch.

• A *Pitta* **pulse** is said to jump like a frog or a crow. It is felt under the middle finger and its quality is strong, bounding, regular and forceful, with a full volume; it feels as if it jumps up forcibly to your finger. The skin may feel warm to the touch and the artery generally feels flexible.

• A *Kapha* **pulse** glides like a swan through the water or an elephant strolling through the jungle. It is deep, slow, soft, regular and slippery, and can be hard to feel because it is deep and not forceful, and because of subcutaneous fat over the artery. The skin may feel cool, thick and soft, and the artery may also feel soft and thick.

Rate (*Vega*)

• *Vata:* **Fast.** In balance the pulse rate is 80 beats per minute. When aggravated, indicating fear or anxiety, it is 80–90. When depleted, it could be as low as 60, as *Prana* (life force) is weak.

• *Pitta:* **Medium.** In balance it is 75–85. When aggravated, indicating fever or inflammation, it is above 85.

• *Kapha:* **Slow.** In balance it is 60–70. When aggravated, indicating lethargy, slow metabolism, and congestion, it is below 60.

The pulse can reveal much about the patient, not only physically, but also mentally and emotionally.

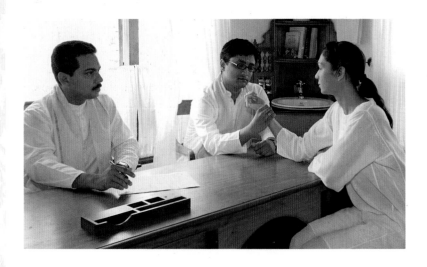

Some very 'fit' people have a slow heart rate. In Ayurvedic terms, this is because they have weakened *Rasa dhatu* (plasma tissue) and this can weaken the heart, manifesting in a slow pulse.

Rhythm (*Tala*)

The rhythm of the pulse should be continually regular and rhythmical.

- **Regular**: *Vata* is balanced.

- **Irregular**: *Vata* is aggravated.

- **Regularly irregular**: *Vata* and *Kapha* are out of balance as beats are missed regularly, such as every fifth beat. *Kapha* gives some stability to the irregular *Vata* nature. It could mean that an excess of *Kapha* is blocking the movement of *Vata*.

- **Irregularly irregular**: *Vata* and *Pitta* are both out of balance. This could mean that *Vata* and *Pitta* compound each other's mobile and moving qualities, or that *Vata* or *Pitta* is obstructing the flow of

Vata. This could be the case in atrial fibrillation.

Level

The flow of the pulse tells us about the quality and quantity of *Prana*, and its force should be equal at every level when a patient is healthy. There are three basic pulse levels. 'Deep' denotes the quality and quantity of *Ojas* (strength) and reflects the deeper nutrition in the tissues. 'Middle' relates to the central nutrition in the organs. 'Superficial' relates to the vitality in the tissues and reflects the state of *Agni*.

- If the pulse is weak in the superficial level, but strong at the deep level, it means that *Agni* is weak from either excess *Vata* or stagnation of *Kapha* and not enough to raise the *Prana* to the surface of the pulse.

- If the pulse is superficially strong and rapid, it may indicate high *Pitta* and *Agni* in the *Rasa dhatu*, with signs of fever or infection.

• When the pulse is superficially weak, it can mean there is a deficiency of *Vata* and *Pitta*, and that *Agni*, *Ojas* and *Prana* are depleted.

• When the pulse is weak in all three positions, it indicates that *Agni*, *Ojas* and *Prana* are weak and that *Vata*, *Pitta* and *Kapha* are depleted or obstructed.

Determining *Prakruti* and *Vikruti*

Prakruti is felt at the deep level, whereas *Vikruti* is felt at the superficial level. If the pulses are the same at both deep and surface level, it means you are in good health and that your *Vikruti* is the same as your *Prakruti*. If there is a difference between the deep and the superficial pulses, it means your *doshas* are not balanced. You can assess the deep level by pressing the pulse firmly until you can no longer feel your pulse. Slowly raise your fingers and, as the pulse returns, this is the deep

level revealing the *Prakruti*. Continue to raise your fingers, and the pulse that you feel just before you lose it altogether is your superficial pulse.

Strength (*Bala*)

Bala is the 'strength' of the pulse felt under the fingers at different levels. There are three basic forces to the pulse: strong, medium and weak.

• A strong pulse reflects any excess or displaced *Agni* and indicates high *Pitta*.

• A medium pulse indicates balanced *Agni* and *Ojas* and is generally found in balanced *Kapha*.

• A weak pulse reflects a depleted *Agni* and *Ojas* and indicates high *Vata*.

Volume (*Akruti*)

The volume of blood in the pulse is felt as the uplift of the pulse wave to the finger, which relates to the systolic blood pressure as the heart beat pushes the blood

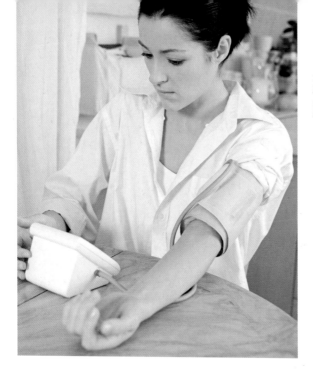

The volume of the blood in the pulse relates to the systolic blood pressure.

into the arteries. It tells us about the quality of *Prana Vata* and *Ranjaka Pitta*.

- Low volume: *Vata*
- Medium volume: *Pitta*
- High volume: *Kapha*

Toxins (*Ama*)

Generally speaking, the presence of *Ama* is indicated by a sluggish and slippery pulse, which may also be hard, heavy and tense. This means that it is hard to the touch, but slips away from the fingers if you exert more pressure. It will be slow, deep and sluggish in *Sama Kapha*; fast, bounding, forceful and tense in *Sama Pitta*; and very fast or very slow with tension and weakness in *Sama Vata* – these being the *Ama* conditions of *Kapha*, *Pitta* and *Vata* respectively.

Tongue diagnosis (*Jibha pariksha*)

Using a mirror and, in a good light, open your mouth and extend your tongue – not to its maximum extension, but just to a comfortable stretch. A normal tongue is of medium size (in relation to overall body size) and a fresh, pink colour with a thin, moist coating without any markings.

Shape and form

• *Vata:* A *Vata* tongue reflects the dry, rough, mobile, light and deficient qualities of *Vata*. It may be small, thin, dry, cracked, deviated and quivering. It is likely to be pale, due to low *Agni*, and to have indentations or scalloped, dry edges, indicating poor absorption of nutrients. It could be a bluish colour, due to stagnation of circulating *Vyana Vata* (see page 56 from cold. There may be dark or black discolorations. It could be depressed at the back of the tongue, indicating low *Ojas*, and cracked at the front, indicating lung dryness. *Vata*-predominant people are often anxious about extending their tongue and find it difficult to extend it very far. An extremely short tongue is a sign of low *Ojas*.

• *Pitta:* A *Pitta* tongue reflects the sharp and penetrating, liquid, hot properties of *Pitta*. It is characteristically long, narrow, pointed and extended forcefully. Due to heat in the body it is likely to be red or to have red spots, raised red papillae, swollen and red edges or a red tip. Redness of the tongue indicates high *Pitta* in *Rasa* or the *Rakta dhatu* (see page 66); if it looks orange it means high *Pitta* in the *Rakta dhatu*, or it could be purple-red due to high *Pitta* condensing *Rasa* and *Rakta dhatu*, resulting in viscous and sluggish circulation.

• *Kapha:* A *Kapha* tongue reflects the unctuous, fluid, soft, slimy, smooth and cold qualities of *Kapha*. It tends to be large, wide, swollen, thick, soft, wet or covered in saliva. Low digestive fire is indicated by a pale tongue and wet, scalloped edges. There may be a swollen tip indicating heart congestion, or it could be swollen in the centre, indicating lung congestion. The tongue could also be pale due to poor circulation or pale blue, due to congestive heart disorders caused by aggravated

A healthy tongue looks a fresh pink colour and has a thin, moist coating.

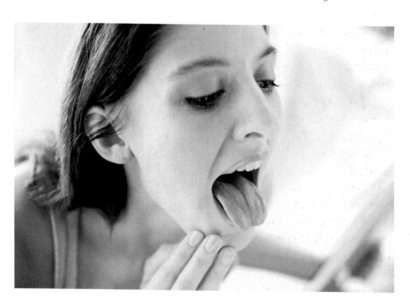

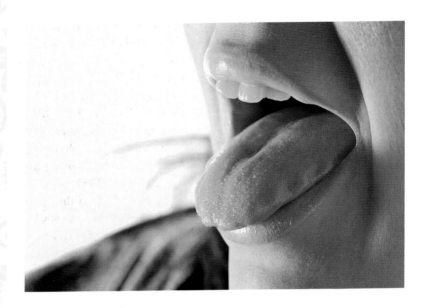

Avalambaka Kapha (see page 62). The *Kapha* tongue can be so large and swollen that it looks as though it could be too large to put back in the mouth!

Certain substances like coffee, tobacco, flavoured drinks and coloured sweets can discolour the tongue coating. Drinking hot drinks and eating spicy meals can make the tongue's body redder. Antibiotics can give the tongue a

The tooth marks around the edge of this tongue indicate poor absorption of nutrients.

thick coating or a shiny-peeled appearance.

Coating

Tongue coatings can be many different colours, depths and textures, each conveying a different message about the internal state of the body. They can be white, yellow and even black, indicating the type and location of *Ama* in the body. The changes in the tongue coating are an easy way to tell if the treatment you are following is having a beneficial effect and the toxins are clearing.

• *Vata:* Dry, thin and white, generally in the *Vata* area at the back of the tongue, which represents the colon.

• *Pitta:* Yellow. If it is also greasy it indicates a mixture of high *Pitta* and *Ama*. If yellow and dry, it means a mixture of *Pitta* and *Vata*. There may be a red, glossy, shiny tongue with no coating, due to intense heat 'burning' the coating away as a sign of excess *Pitta*. This would indicate a weak and deficient condition caused by the over-fast metabolism of nutrients. The coating is likely to be more in the middle of the tongue, which is associated with the stomach and small intestines. The sides of the

tongue relate to the liver, and many *Pitta* imbalances are also seen here.

• *Kapha:* White, thick, wet, clear. If the coating is thick, white and greasy, it means a mixture of *Kapha* and *Ama*. If pale yellow, it indicates a mixture of *Kapha* and *Pitta*. The coating is likely to be clearest on either side of the midline of the tongue in the part associated with the lungs, chest and heart. If there is a lot of *Kapha* and *Ama*, then a thick, greasy coating may cover the whole tongue.

Central crack

A central crack in the tongue reflects the flow of *Prana* through the heart or spine. If the crack goes to the tip of the tongue, it may mean a congenital heart weakness. A deviated crack can indicate back problems. A crack may also appear due to excess *Kapha* causing the two sides of the tongue to swell.

Chapter 10: The principles of Ayurvedic treatment (*Chikitsa*)

Ayurveda is such a comprehensive system that if you follow its recommendations you have the potential to enjoy the vibrant state of health that is the basis of all four goals of life (see page 25) – including the ultimate goal of *Moksha,* which is liberation.

Indications of good health

According to Ayurveda, the signs and symptoms of a healthy person are:

- *Samadosha*: the *doshas* must be in equilibrium
- *Samagnischa*: *Agni* (digestive fire) must be in a balanced state to prevent a build-up of toxins
- *Samadhatumala*: the seven *dhatus* (tissues) and *malas* (waste products) must be functioning properly to ensure that *Ama*

(toxins) is cleared from the system
- **Balance**: the sensory organs, motor organs, mind and Atman must be in a balanced state.

These are reflected in the following signs of good health:
- A healthy appetite and a balanced desire for food, without cravings
- Appreciation of the flavour of food, and feeling satisfied after eating
- Good digestion without any signs of discomfort
- Clear voice
- Absence of any pain or discomfort
- Appropriate length and quality of sleep: six to eight hours per night

A healthy appetite without food cravings is a sign of good health.

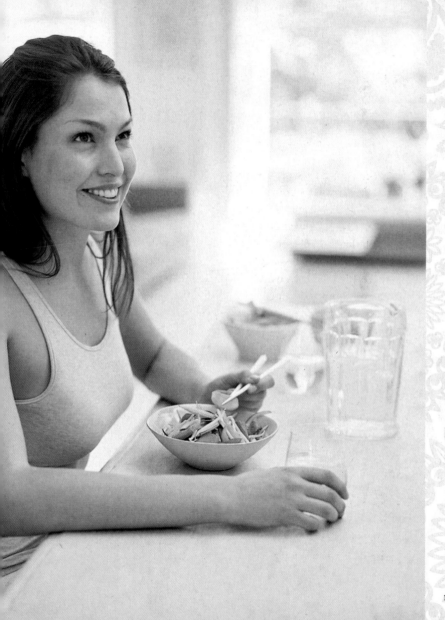

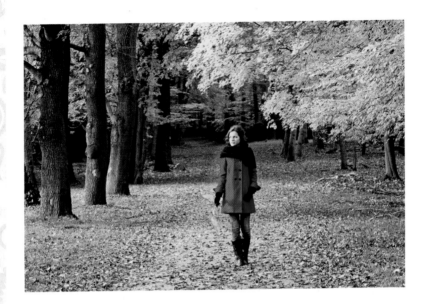

Good energy and stamina are another indicator of good health.

- Clear complexion
- Regular elimination of stool, urine and sweat
- Constant energy with good stamina and the ability to exercise
- Enthusiasm for life
- Balanced emotions: neither too happy with success nor too sad in times of difficulty
- Being compassionate, generous and calm.

The aim of Ayurvedic treatment (_Chikitsa_) is to balance the _doshas, dhatus_ and _malas_. To do this it is important to ensure a healthy digestive fire, eliminate any toxins, clear obstructions in the _srotas_ (channels) and balance _Prana_ (life force), _Teja_ (radiant energy) and _Ojas_ (strength) (see page 266).

This should be followed by rejuvenation therapy (*Rasayana*, see Chapter 18) to enhance continued good health and vitality.

Addressing the roots of disease

The wisdom of Ayurveda emphasizes the importance of addressing the roots of health and disease, rather than the thousands of disease symptoms that arise from them. It is an approach that is simple without being simplistic, and can be grasped by any of us who want to maximize our healing potential through an understanding of ourselves and the universe around us.

First you need to assess your *Prakruti* and your *Vikruti* – that is, your basic constitution and current *doshic* imbalance. Full health and well-being are only possible when the *doshas* work harmoniously together. Each person displays a varying combination of the three *doshas*,

and if you understand your basic constitution you will know your weaknesses and inherited tendencies and can then adopt the right diet and lifestyle to keep you in the best possible health. This is the ideal way to prevent depletion of your health and strength and consequent ill health.

If you consult a practitioner, he/she will take a detailed case history and examine you, paying attention to your build, skin and hair type, the temperature of your body, your digestion and bowel function and your temperament – all of which point to more profound aspects of your condition. Tongue and pulse diagnosis are valuable diagnostic tools used by Ayurvedic practitioners. Once your *doshic* balance, the state of the *dhatus* and *malas* have been diagnosed and the causes of any imbalances established, the dietary and lifestyle advice are relatively straightforward. Herbs will be prescribed.

Ayurvedic treatments

Treatment that you can use at home, and that most Ayurvedic practitioners in the West employ, is known as palliative therapy (*Shamana*) – as opposed to *Panchakarma* or purification therapy (which is known as *Shodhana*), conducted in special clinics.

Shamana traditionally employs six main techniques to balance the *dosha*s, *dhatu*s and *mala*s, raise *Agni* and clear *Ama*:

1 Reduction therapy (*Langhana*) for cleaning excesses of *Ama/dosha*s

2 Tonifying (*Brimhana*) is used where there is a deficiency, using sweet and nourishing tonics (*Rasayanas*) in the form of foods and herbs

3 Drying (*Rukshana*) to clear excess fluid, using diuretic and astringent herbs

4 Oil application (*Snehana*) to reduce dryness, using oils and massage as well as soothing herbs

5 Fomentation or therapeutic sweating (*Swedana*) to dispel coldness, stiffness and heat that has accumulated in the body, using steam and diaphoretic herbs (see page 192)

6 Astringent (*Stambhana*) herbs to constrict channels and reduce the excess flow of fluids, such as diarrhoea or bleeding.

Vagbhata, a famous Ayurvedic physician from about the 7th century CE, created two broad categories of treatment: *Langhana*, meaning 'reduction', and *Brimhana*, meaning 'tonification'.

1 *Langhana*

This reduces, breaks down and detoxifies the body, cleansing it of excess accumulations, toxins and impaired *doshas*. It is further subdivided into *Langhana* proper, or cleansing (both *Shamana* and *Shodhana*, see detoxification on page 206); *Rukshana*, or drying; and *Swedana*, or sweating. *Shamana* comprises most of the everyday cleansing practices that can be done at home on a regular basis. They can also be used in preparation for *Shodhana* or *Panchakarma*, and can be divided into the following:

• *Dipana*: kindling the digestive fire using pungent, hot, drying herbs to stimulate *Agni*

• *Pachana*: clearing *Ama* toxins and undigested food residues (see detoxification on page 217)

• *Vrat* or *Kshud nigraha*: fasting (see detoxification on page 213)

• *Trsna* or *Trn nigraha*: fasting from, or reducing, fluid intake (particularly recommended for excess *Kapha*, but only to be done on the advice of a practitioner)

• *Vyayama*: exercise and yoga

• *Atapa*: lightening, drying and reducing the *doshas* by sitting in the sun and raising the metabolism

• *Maruta*: lightening and drying the body by sitting in the wind and through breathing practices (see *Pranayama* on page 278).

2 *Brimhana*

This is used to nourish, strengthen, enrich and fortify the body and generally follows *Langhana*. It involves the use of nourishing and rejuvenating foods and tonic herbs. It is further subdivided into *Brimhana* (diet and herbs), *Snehana* (oil application) and *Stambhana* (astringency). *Brimhana* diet and herbs are intended to increase

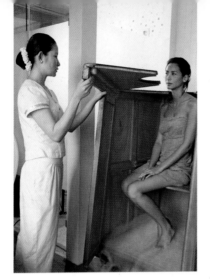

A sweat box is used after oil massage and is very good for reducing Vata.

weight and strength and to increase *Kapha* in depleted and debilitated people. They are particularly useful during convalescence, for people who are too thin, weak and rundown from excess *Vata*.

3 Rukshana

This is the intake of foods and herbs that have diuretic properties to clear excess water from the body, in conjunction with dry massage using powdered herbs. It is particularly useful for excess *Kapha* manifesting in diseases such as diabetes and obesity.

4 Snehana

This is the use of oils and fats in the form of ghee (clarified butter), both internally and externally to increase lubrication and nutrition. It has a calming, grounding and stabilizing effect, physically and mentally, and is particularly recommended for disturbances of *Vata* and, to a lesser extent, *Pitta*.

5 Swedana

This comprises therapies that increase body heat and cause sweating, and they are particularly good for excess *Vata*. They include the external application of dry heat or steam, or taking warming herbs such as ginger, cinnamon or Trikatu. These herbs are also good for *Kapha*.

6 Stambhana

This is done less frequently and involves using drying and

constricting herbs to reduce blood, lymph and other excess fluids in the body. It is particularly used for *Pitta*-type bleeding disorders and diarrhoea.

Addressing imbalances

There is a variety of different ways to remedy imbalances of the *doshas* and *dhatus*, which all involve enhancing our relationship with the world around us. Ayurveda uses herbal medicines and wholesome foods and addresses every aspect of daily living.

The herbs, diet and lifestyle advocated for each individual patient will vary, according their effect on the three *doshas* and the seven *dhatus*.

STRATEGIES FOR TREATMENT

The strategies for treatment are generally as follows:

- Treatment of the *doshas* (see page 224)
- Treatment of *Agni* (see page 198)
- Treatment of the *dhatus* (see page 250)
- Treatment of the specific disease (*Vyadhi*)
- Detoxification and clearing the *Ama* with *Ama Pachana* (see page 217) or *Panchakarma*; pacification of the disease and clearing *Ama* with *Shamana* (see detoxification on page 206)
- Treatment of the *gunas* (three qualities) by increasing *Sattva* (clarity and harmony) and reducing *Rajas* (energy and action) and *Tamas* (decay and inertia) (see page 227)
- Rejuvenation with tonics (see *Rasayana* on page 373).

Balancing excess and deficiency

Ayurveda classifies conditions of the *doshas*, *dhatus*, *malas* and *Agni* as involving excess, deficiency or vitiation.

• **Excess (*Vridhi*)** could mean too much heat, cold, dryness, dampness, wind, mucus, *Ama* (toxins), *mala*, or excesses of *doshas* and *dhatus*; for instance, *Pitta* is increased in hot, sunny weather, causing prickly heat and irritation.

• **Deficiency (*Kshaya*)** could mean too little heat, moisture, physical strength, digestive energy, mental resilience, or deficient states of *doshas* and *dhatus*; for example, deficient bone tissue (*Asthi dhatu*) may lead to osteoporosis.

• **Vitiation or impairment (*Prakopa*)** means that the *doshas*, *dhatus* and *Agni* are disturbed and deranged; for instance, *Vata* is often disturbed by a storm and this can cause insomnia, while *Pitta* can be disturbed and cause intense jealousy or depression.

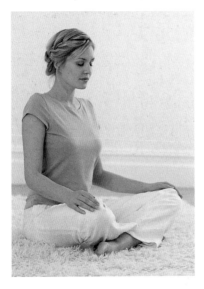

Factors of similar nature to health, including yoga and meditation, improve health.

'Like increases like', but opposites attract

One of the tenets of Ayurvedic treatment is to enhance health by developing factors of similar nature to it (*Samanya*) and by reducing factors of contrary nature (*Vishesha*). Factors of similar nature to health, such as rest, good food or meditation, will increase health. Those of an opposite nature, such as overwork, alcohol, bad diet or stress, will detract from it.

However, there is also the idea that health imbalances are corrected by their opposite: a condition of excess heat is corrected by using cooling foods such as coconut milk, and herbs such as neem and andrographis; and a cold, dry condition of the joint is alleviated by application of warm oils such as ginger.

Excess pathologies are treated using substances with qualities that are opposite to the disease, while deficient pathologies are treated using herbs with similar properties.

Building an Ayurvedic herbal formula

A recommended method for composing a herbal prescription is to follow the order in which disease needs to be treated, using one or two herbs for each aspect of the treatment as follows:

• Herbs for *Agni*
• Herbs to clear *Ama*
• Herbs to balance the *doshas*
• Herbs to balance the *dhatus*
• Herbs for the specific disease.

You may also want to use herbs to increase *Sattwa* and balance the *gunas* (see Chapter 15 for herb profiles).

For example, for the treatment of arthritis with aggravated *Vata* in the bone tissue with a low digestive fire and *Ama*, you could use the following herbs:

• For the *Agni*: ginger, cardamom
• For the *Ama*: asafoetida, Triphala
• For the *dosha*: ashwagandha, bala
• For the *dhatu*: frankincense, guggulu
• For the disease: turmeric, gotu kola.

Chapter 11: **Detoxification**

In the Ayurvedic tradition, detoxification and rejuvenation (*Rasayana*) represent the primary approach to maintaining positive health of mind and body. Regular periods of detoxification can help protect you from, and treat, a variety of health problems, increase energy and vitality and promote a sense of well-being.

The process of detoxification

The whole process of Ayurvedic detoxification first involves clearing the *Ama* (toxins), then balancing the disturbed *doshas* and finally nourishment of the tissues that have been damaged through toxicity and any resultant illness (*Rasayana*).

Toxins are substances that are potentially harmful to the body: they lower our defences, predisposing us to ill health and speeding up the ageing process. Free radicals (molecules that cause tissue damage) develop due to the accumulation of toxins in the body. Research points to the role of free radicals in the development of many degenerative diseases and immune problems such as cancer. Toxins themselves are a product of our lifestyle, our digestion, our diet, the environment and our emotional patterns.

Taking ginger tea first thing in the morning is recommended for detoxification.

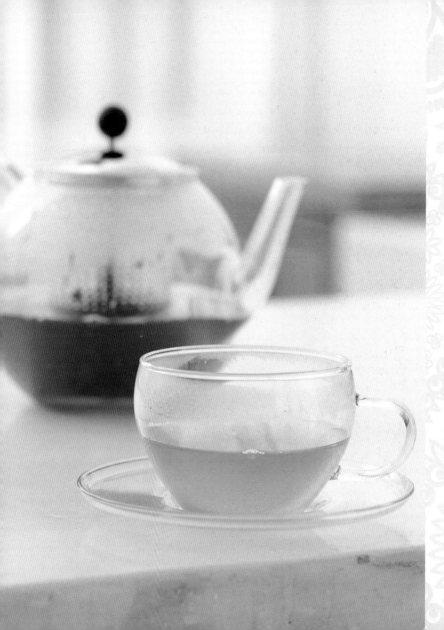

Agni and *Ama*

One of the main tenets of Ayurveda is that good digestion is vital for optimum health, and incomplete or disordered digestion can be a major contributor to the development of disease.

When *Agni* (digestive fire) is strong, our food is digested and assimilated into its fundamental five elements (see page 28) and then these are absorbed to nourish our cells and

tissues (see *dhatus* on page 64). When we are healthy, any of the digested food that is not useful to the body is eliminated via the three pathways of elimination (*malas*):

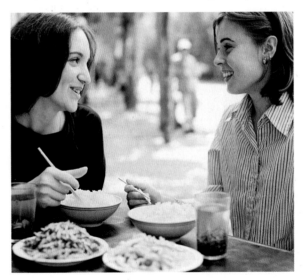

When our Agni *is good our food is digested and assimilated to nourish our cells and tissues.*

urine, faeces and sweat (see *malas* on page 75).

Our internal environment is governed by the three *doshas* (see page 32), which are constantly reacting to the external environment. The wrong diet and lifestyle for your *dosha* or for the season, incompatible food combinations (such as milk and fish, melons and grain, yoghurt and meat or cooked honey), repressed emotions and stress can all change the balance of our *doshas* and affect our *Agni*. The poorly digested food ferments and produces *Ama*, which enters the bloodstream and circulates throughout the body, clogging the channels. *Ama* is increased by eating too much, when we are stressed or before the previous meal has been digested, by going to sleep on a full stomach or by eating foods that are leftover, processed, old or fermented. If accumulated toxicity becomes well established, it will slowly affect *Prana* (vital life energy), *Ojas* (strength and immunity), and *Tejas*

(cellular metabolic energy) and will result in disease. The symptoms that result from this could be interpreted as our body's effort to eliminate toxins. *Ama* is the basic cause of all disease.

It is possible to have *Vata*, *Pitta* or *Kapha* imbalances, either with or without *Ama*. When *Ama* is associated with one of the three *doshas*, it becomes known as *Sama* and the symptoms vary according to the *dosha* that is involved:

- **Sama Kapha** is indicated by indigestion and mucus congestion.

- **Sama Pitta** is indicated by indigestion, hyperacidity and diarrhoea, fever or skin conditions.

- **Sama Vata** occurs with tiredness, abdominal distension, gas and constipation.

If there is toxicity in the body, the right foods and herbs cannot be properly utilized by the body and it is hard to balance the *doshas* until

Ama has been removed. Then more specific measures for balancing the *doshas* and nourishing the cells and tissues can be effective. So the first stage of treatment with Ayurveda normally involves some degree of detoxification.

The channels of circulation (*srotas*)

The body contains innumerable channels through which nutrients, the basic tissue elements, *doshas* and *malas* (waste products) circulate (see the *srotas* on page 78). If *Ama* is produced over a long period of time, it can leave the digestive tract, travel to a weak area elsewhere in the body and settle there. It creates blockages in the *srotas* and disrupts the flow of nourishment to the cells and tissues, and the excretion of wastes through the pathways of elimination. The metabolism of the tissues is subsequently affected, predisposing us to the onset of disease in the affected part. As well as *Ama*, excess *doshas* and *malas* can be moved by *Vata* and accumulate in the *srotas*. Blockage here is considered the main cause of disease in Ayurveda.

In addition the accumulated toxins in the gut block the function of *Agni*, compromising the digestion, absorption and assimilation of nutrients, causing tiredness and depletion and poor nutrient supply to all the tissues.

Types of toxins

There are three different types of toxins that can disrupt normal functioning of the *srotas*: *Ama*, *Amavisha* and *Garvisha*.

Ama

Ama – the waste product of incomplete digestion – is the most common type of toxin. It is described as heavy, thick, cold, sticky and foul-smelling, while *Agni* is light, clear, hot and pure. Incompletely digested food materials ferment and set up an internal environment that supports the growth of pathogenic (disease-

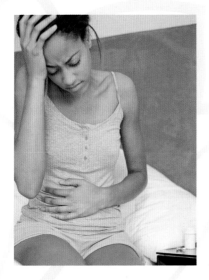

Toxins in the gut can wreak havoc with our immune systems and predispose us to food allergies and autoimmune disease.

through straightforward detoxification processes that you can follow at home. By enhancing *Agni* through dietary changes and taking Ayurvedic herbs, the digestive system itself can burn off simple *Ama* and clear it from the body (for more on this, see page 214).

Amavisha

Amavisha is a more reactive form of toxicity that forms when *Ama* settles in one part of the body for a long time and mixes there with the sub-*doshas*, *dhatus* or *malas*. *Amavisha* causes the *srotas* to become hardened and dried with toxins, which then causes damage to the *srotas*.

causing) bacteria, yeasts and parasites. Endotoxins (toxins in the gut) irritate the gut lining, causing small holes in the gut wall (known as 'leaky gut syndrome'), which allow molecules of undigested and partially digested food, as well as toxins, through the gut wall. These wreak havoc with our immune systems and predispose us to food allergies and autoimmune disease.

Blockage of the *srotas* with simple *Ama* is relatively easy to remove,

A toxic mixture of *Ama*, *Amavisha* and *Shleshaka Kapha* (a sub-*dosha* of *Kapha* concerned with maintaining proper fluid balance and lubrication of the body) can combine together, causing excess moisture, which in turn causes *Vyana Vata* (the sub-*dosha* of *Vata* concerned with circulation) to accelerate its drying effect, causing this toxic, sticky sludge to adhere to the walls of the *srotas*. They become dry, inflexible and narrowed, with the risk of ensuing blockage. This is the Ayurvedic explanation for the development of atherosclerosis and its associated problems of heart disease and strokes.

Removing this deeper and chronic type of toxicity is a more complex problem and necessitates certain preparatory treatments before detoxification, to lubricate and soften the stubborn toxins and enable their removal. This is to prevent further damage to the *srotas* by over-stringent detoxification. Internal and external oil treatment to loosen toxins is therefore recommended before clearing *Ama*. Taking ghee internally and using warm sesame oil massage is recommended (see page 246).

Garvisha

This third type of *Ama*, which causes more serious damage to the *srotas*, is the most problematic. *Garvisha* involves the absorption into the body of environmental toxins such as chemicals, preservatives, poisons, air and water pollution, genetically engineered foods, synthetics and chemicals in clothing, synthetic drugs, chemicals in household cleansers, and heavy metals such as lead and asbestos. It also includes toxins from spoiled foods. Most of today's environmental toxins accumulate in the fatty tissues of the body and are implicated in a range of health problems, including hormone disruption, immune-system deficiency, allergies, diseases of the liver and skin, different types of cancer, neurological problems and reproductive disorders.

When the harmful combination of *Shleshaka Kapha*, *Vyana Vata*, *Amavisha* and *Ama* becomes augmented by *Garvisha*, it can manifest in illness such as

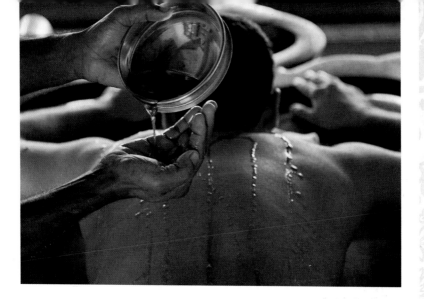

ulcerative colitis, multiple sclerosis and other autoimmune diseases. At this stage, in-house deeper detoxification in the shape of *Panchakarma* (see Chapter 17) is recommended.

Preventative measures

Prevention is the key to health. Follow the diet and lifestyle for your *dosha*, exercise every day to improve your digestion and elimination, do a daily *Abhyanga* (warm-oil massage) to flush out toxins through the skin, drink

Internal and external oil treatment to loosen toxins is recommended before clearing chronic toxicity.

herbal teas suitable for your imbalances, and meditate every day to remove stress. In terms of lifestyle changes, during a period of cleansing all activities that are *Prajnaya paradha* ('crimes against wisdom') should be avoided. This includes smoking, recreational drugs and activities that are habitual, such as the use of coffee, alcohol and white sugar.

Seasonal times to detox

Ayurvedic seasonal routines and dietary guidelines play an important part in preventative health (see Chapter 7), too. By following simple guidelines, you can help mitigate the toxins that accumulate due to seasonal changes.

A short period of detoxification at least once a year is recommended, but not for pregnant women, nursing mothers, children or patients with chronic degenerative diseases, cancer or tuberculosis. If your health is generally good and you probably have an imbalance of one or other *dosha* and simple *Ama*, you can do a good detox following the methods of *Shamana* (see page 206).

If you suffer from more chronic health problems you may have some degree of *Amavisha* or *Garvisha* and it is better to consult an Ayurvedic practitioner for guidance on specific recommendations.

In winter the *srotas* contract, inhibiting the free flow of nutrients

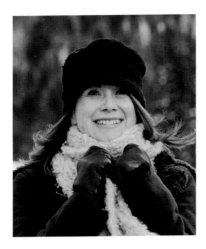

Winter, when the srotas *contract, is not the best time to do a detox.*

BEST DETOX TIMES

The ideal times to undergo gentle cleansing and restore balance to the body are as follows:

- *Vata*: at the end of summer before autumn sets in – the crossover time just before *Vata* is aggravated
- *Pitta*: in late spring, just before the summer, when *Pitta* becomes aggravated
- *Kapha*: at the end of winter, before spring begins.

and wastes and making it harder for the body to release toxins. During the transition between the seasons our *Agni* fluctuates, which can cause *Ama* to accumulate, even if you are careful about your diet and routine. For this reason it is a good idea to do a detox or *Panchakarma* during each change of seasons, particularly in the spring when the body is naturally detoxifying. The changing seasons also predispose us to accumulations of specific *doshas*, so cleansing at this time can be helpful in reducing the accumulation of *Vata*, *Pitta* or *Kapha*.

There is some consensus between East and West regarding cleansing toxins in spring, for there is a tradition in Britain to use herbs such as dandelions and nettles to do a spring detox. During spring, toxins that have accumulated through the winter begin to surface. This is the best time to clear them in order to avoid illness during the summer season. Once cleansed, the body is ready for spontaneous healing even without medication; and if medication is given it has a better chance of flowing to its target sites, leading to greater efficacy with fewer side-effects.

Methods of detoxification

As we have seen, there are two levels of detoxification treatment. The first is known as *Shamana* or palliative therapy and involves enhancing digestion and elimination, while the second is the stronger purification therapy known as *Shodhana*.

Shamana is a slow and gentle method of detoxification, best suited to home treatment. It can be employed as part of a mild detox for those not needing, or unable, to undergo deeper cleansing. When instigated from time to time, or over a period of time, palliative therapy can be as effective as *Shodhana* and is the method of detoxification that is discussed below. There are three stages to this process – preparation, detoxification and nourishing – each of which is described in detail.

Shodhana or *Panchakarma* (see Chapter 17) is more deep-acting and necessitates in-patient care in special therapy centres. There are some existing *Panchakarma* centres in the West, but otherwise this treatment is generally only available in India and Sri Lanka.

1 Preparation

Preparation is a vital part of an Ayurvedic detox programme. It is important to take into account each individual's balance of the *doshas* (*Vikruti*), the state of their *srotas*, their *Agni* (digestive fire), and whether high, low, irregular or balanced, and the type of toxins present, to determine the best detox procedures and whether *Shamana* is sufficient or *Panchakarma* would be better.

To prepare the body, it is important first to balance *Agni*. If *Agni* is overly high, you need to take herbs or eat foods to reduce it. If it is low, you need to take *Agni*-enhancing foods and herbs. If *Vata* has disturbed *Agni* and caused it to become irregular, it is important to balance it.

As far as your *doshic* balance is concerned, if you have more *Kapha* and are overweight, you will need a *Kapha*-pacifying diet and more warming herbs. If you have a *Pitta* imbalance, you will need a *Pitta*-pacifying diet and herbs to clear heat and cleanse the liver.

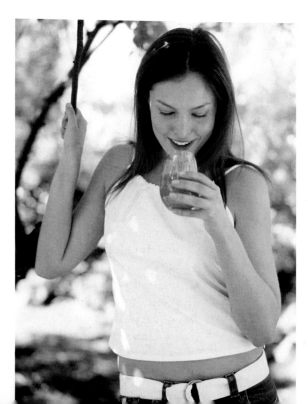

Freshly juiced fruits can form part of a detoxifying diet.

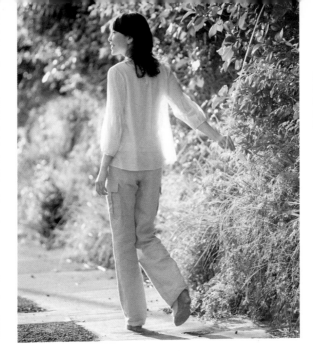

It is recommended to take a walk early in the morning when the atmosphere is Sattvic.

For a thin person with *Vata* aggravation, a lubricating and nurturing diet and herbs are needed, as the *srotas* are likely to have become dry, causing the toxins to dry and stick to the *srota* walls. The Charaka Samhita explains that in an underweight person the *malas* (wastes) provide a type of strength and support in the *srotas*; lubrication and nurture are important before detoxification, so

that you can tolerate the process without inviting risk of depletion, fatigue or mental disturbance. (For more on balancing the *doshas*, see page 226.)

Generally speaking, preparation should be done over 14–30 days, or even up to two months, and during this time it is important to do the following:

- **Rest**: Ensure you get enough rest, keeping regular hours of sleeping

208

and waking, ideally going to bed at 10 p.m. and waking at 6 a.m. Staying up late and sleeping late in the morning can increase the stagnation of toxins in the *srotas*.

- **Reduce stress**: Practising meditation and *Pranayama* (breathing exercises) regularly will help to reduce stress and enhance the cleansing process, especially of mental and emotional *Ama*.

- **Gentle exercise**: Exercise such as yoga and walking improves the digestion and elimination and helps clear toxins from the body. Walking for 20–30 minutes daily, if possible, while breathing deeply, purifies the respiratory system, oxygenates it and supplies the cells and tissues with cleansing *Prana* (life force), as does *Pranayama*. Walking in the early morning is especially recommended when the atmosphere is *Sattvic* (clear and uplifting).

- **Warm oil massage** (*Abhyanga*): This is central to detoxification in Ayurveda. Massaging the whole body with oils is best done every day, either on rising or in the evening before going to bed. Leave the oil on for 10–15 minutes before soaking in a warm bath or shower. *Abhyanga* loosens toxins under the skin and in the outer part of the body, encouraging them to flow into the digestive tract, where they can easily be eliminated through the bowel. Massage is very relaxing and helps to increase resilience to stress. It also enhances the circulation. Oils can be chosen according to your *doshic* type. Sesame oil is used fairly generally, and herbs or essential oils added to it will help it penetrate the surface of the skin and reach the deeper layers and tissues, purifying and nourishing the *srotas* of the skin. You can also drop a blend of essential oils of niaouli, sandalwood and eucalyptus

AYURVEDIC DIAGNOSIS AND TREATMENT

added to sesame oil (two drops of essential oil per 5 ml of sesame oil) into your bath to draw out the toxins.

- **Take care of your digestion**: Throughout the year, and especially while detoxifying, it is important to take good care of your digestive fire and not eat in a way that will increase *Ama* accumulation (see page 122).

2 Detoxification

A healthy diet is one of the most important tools for preventing and reducing *Ama* accumulation, and when doing a home detox it is best to follow an *Ama*-reducing diet for up to several weeks, depending on the degree of toxicity. I generally do three or four weeks of this twice a year.

Ama-reducing diet

This diet involves eating:
- Freshly prepared foods, which are nutritious and appetizing

- Light foods that are easy to digest, such as rice, vegetable soup and lentils; also freshly baked flatbreads, grains such as barley and basmati rice, with plenty of organic, freshly steamed or lightly sautéed vegetables or freshly juiced fruits

- Mung-bean soup, which pacifies all three *doshas* and is nutritious, yet easy to digest

- Warm and cooked foods, which are easier to digest than raw, hard foods; seeds can be eaten in small amounts

- White meat, turkey or chicken and fish, which are preferable to red meats.

Certain foods are especially helpful during cleansing:
- **Vegetables**: Eat lots of cooked leafy green vegetables with mild spices. Beetroot, radishes, artichokes, cabbage, broccoli, spirulina, chlorell and seaweed

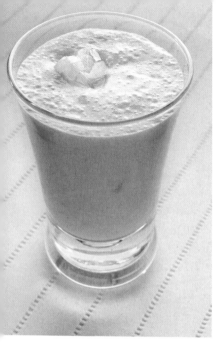

Lassi is a mixture of yoghurt and water with added spices to enhance its digestion.

small helpings of rice are recommended. Kanji, which is made by boiling rice with lots of water, is excellent for flushing toxins out through the urine.

- **Lassi**: Made by combining fresh yoghurt with water and digestive spices, this is an excellent lunchtime beverage.

- **Kefir**: This cultured-milk beverage is made by inoculating milk with kefir grains, a mixture of yeasts and bacteria that will sour the milk slightly, creating a drink that is almost like liquid yoghurt. People who prefer not to use dairy may also make kefir from plant or nut milks, such as coconut or almond milk. The beneficial strains of yeast in kefir help to eliminate pathogenic yeasts in the gut by penetrating the mucosal lining where they reside. In

are all excellent detoxifying foods.

- **Spices**: Ginger, turmeric, cumin, coriander, fennel and fenugreek can be added to your meals, as they open up the *srotas* and help clear toxins via the skin, urinary tract, colon and liver.

- **Grains**: Whole grains such as quinoa, barley, amaranth and

ancient Ayurvedic texts, fermented milk was often used to heal digestive disorders, but was always diluted with water.

- **Warm water or herbal teas**: Drink teas such as fennel, lemongrass or mint throughout the day to help flush toxins out of the body through the urine. Ginger tea is an excellent way to raise *Agni* and clear *Ama*. It is best drunk in the morning before breakfast and again before lunch. Ginger tea can also be sipped throughout the day. Hot water and a squeeze of lime makes a good alternative and may be preferable for some palates.

Choose foods according to your body type or imbalances to help regulate your digestive fire (*Agni*) (see Chapter 12).

Minimize foods that increase *Ama* (*Amagenic*):

- Tinned, devitalized, frozen, 'junk' or stale leftovers
- Dairy products
- Refined carbohydrates such as white flour and sugar
- Yeasted breads and dry breads such as crackers
- Fermented foods and drinks, including vinegar, chutneys and pickles
- Cold foods and drinks
- Indigestible foods, such as cheese, red meat, heavy desserts, hard and raw foods such as nuts
- Oily, fried, heavy and salty foods
- Non-organic foods, genetically modified foods, foods grown with chemicals, pesticides and chemical fertilizers, and foods with chemical additives

Try to avoid drugs, which may suppress many of the symptoms of *Ama* build-up, but which may increase the workload of the liver and gut and actually increase the build-up of *Ama* at the same time. It is also important to reduce or avoid alcohol, caffeine, drugs and tobacco, and minimize your exposure to household chemicals and synthetic or petroleum-based products.

Ayurvedic fasting
(*Kshud nigraha*)

Fasting rests the digestion and is an effective way to kindle the digestive fire and burn away accumulated toxins from body and mind. It also improves the bowels, eliminates wind, clears the tongue, sweetens the breath, makes the body feel light, and improves mental clarity and overall health. Regular short-term fasting is preferable to infrequent, long-term fasting, which can be depleting and lead to *doshic* imbalance.

When determining the appropriate type and length of a fast, it is important to take into account your constitution, digestive strength, level of *Ama* and overall vitality. For growing children, pregnant women, those who are depleted, thin or undernourished, the elderly or

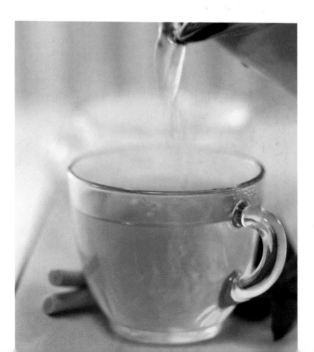

Drink teas of fennel, mint, lemongrass or ginger to help flush out toxins.

chronically ill, complete fasting from all food is not recommended, although reduction of foods when acutely unwell is very natural, and often at these times one loses all appetite for solid food. *Vata*-predominant people can fast on such occasions on hot liquid soups; *Pitta*-predominant people on fruit juices such as grape/pomegranate or vegetable juices; *Kapha*-predominant people simply on water or herbal teas.

The primary types of fasting in Ayurveda include:
• Consuming light foods only, such as *Kichari* (basmati rice and mung beans/red lentils) and *Kanjee* (barley-water and rice)

• Consuming fruits, vegetables or juices only

• Abstaining from solid foods while drinking water or herbal teas.
   During fasting it is important to get plenty of rest and to try to avoid stress. After your fast, begin eating normally again gradually, slowly working your way up to solid foods. During a detox it is best to avoid strenuous exercise and overtaxing the body.

Throughout the year those with a *Pitta* constitution could fast from solid food once a week for a day; *Kapha* types for a few days a month; while those with high *Vata* are likely to be relatively depleted and are best doing a more moderate *Kichari* fast (see opposite).

Raising the digestive fire (*Agni Deepana*)

Agni is increased by pungent, sour and salty tastes and a small amount of bitter taste. By increasing digestive fire with warming and pungent herbs, *Ama* is 'burned' away, and this is known as *Agni Deepana* (raising digestive fire) and *Ama Pachana* (clearing *Ama*).

The best pungent herbs for raising digestive fire include ginger, cinnamon, black pepper, long pepper, asafoetida, cayenne

KICHARI FAST

A *Kichari* fast for two to four weeks is a pleasant and
tasty way to follow a cleansing diet. *Kichari* can be
eaten at least twice a day, for lunch and supper. If
you eat a different vegetable dish with it and vary
the spices and vegetables that you add, it is not nearly
as boring as it sounds!

½ cup split mung beans (or red lentils)
1 cup basmati rice – i.e. twice as much
rice as mung beans/red lentils
a little ghee (clarified butter)
spices of your choice
salt
vegetables of your choice

Wash the mung beans/red lentils and rice thoroughly.

Melt some ghee in a large pan and add spices such
as fresh ginger, turmeric, black cumin seed, freshly
ground fennel, cumin and coriander.

Add the rice and mung beans and 6 cups water, then
bring to a boil. Turn down to a simmer for 45 minutes
or until the beans/lentils are soft. Add salt to taste.

Add vegetables of your choice either during cooking
or separately at the end.

and mustard, and these are ideal for *Sama Kapha* (*Ama* conditions of *Kapha*), but care needs to be taken with very pungent herbs as they may aggravate excess *Pitta* and *Vata*. Warming herbs and spices, such as cardamom, turmeric, cumin, coriander, basil and fennel, have the same qualities as *Agni*, being hot, dry, light and fragrant.

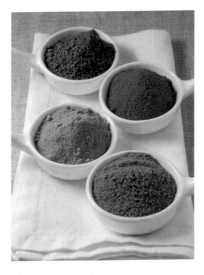

Spices for raising the digestive fire include black pepper, cayenne, turmeric and coriander.

They help to balance *Agni* and *Ama*, and can be used more generally for all three *doshas*.

Well-known formulae (see Chapter 16) for *Agni Deepana* include:

- **Trikatu**: Specifically for low *Agni* and high *Ama*. It reduces *Sama Kapha* and *Sama Vata* and increases *Pitta*. However, it can be helpful for *Sama Pitta* conditions, but in combination with bitter herbs to avoid aggravation of *Pitta* by its hot nature. Take 1–3 gm two to three times daily in warm water.

- **Trikulu** (clove, cinnamon, cardamom): A good digestive and cleansing formula for *Vata* and *Kapha*.

- **Hingwashtaka**: One of the best remedies for *Vata*. Take ½–1 teaspoon in warm water half an hour before eating.

- **Lavanbhaskar**: A good laxative for *Vata*.

- **Talisadi**: This increases *Agni* in *Vata* and *Kapha* conditions. Take it with lime juice or honey.

- **Sitopaladi**: A pleasant-tasting expectorant, which reduces *Kapha* and *Vata*. Take 1–4 gm two to four times daily in a teaspoon of runny honey or ghee.

- **Trisugandhi** (cinnamon, cinnamon leaf, cardamom): A diaphoretic and stimulant formula, recommended for indigestion, poor appetite, wind, distension, to improve digestion and increase *Agni*.

- **Lavangadi**: This reduces *Vata* and *Kapha*, and increases *Agni* and *Pitta*.

Clearing toxins (*Ama Pachana*)

Of the six tastes (see page 124), pungent and bitter tastes are the best for clearing *Ama* from the digestive tract. Sweet, salty and sour tastes increase *Ama*, as they are said to feed toxins. Astringent has a neutral effect; although it can dry up *Ama*, it can hold it in the body by its contracting action.

Bitter-tasting herbs 'scrape' toxins from the tissues and are highly effective in flushing out toxins from the liver, blood, sweat glands and bowels. They are excellent for *Rakta Shodana* or cleansing the liver, which is the main detoxifying organ of the body. It is the liver's job to identify toxins in the nutritive fluid and store them to prevent them going into the blood. If the liver becomes overloaded with chemicals, preservatives or additives from foods or other toxins such as alcohol and drugs, it will no longer be able to work efficiently. Enhancing the function of the liver is a central part of detoxification.

With their cooling effects, bitter herbs can also be used to relieve fever or infections associated with toxicity. They are excellent where there is heat, inflammation, fermentation and toxins in the blood, and for any *Ama* condition related to eating excess sweet or fatty food. They are best for *Sama Pitta* and *Sama Kapha* conditions and can be used in small amounts for long-standing *Sama Vata* conditions.

The best-known Ayurvedic bitters include chiretta, neem, aloe vera, turmeric, guduchi, sariva and manjishta. Western bitters include dandelion root, burdock, milk thistle, gentian and dock root. Formulae such as Tikta (a combination of bitter herbs) and Sudarshan or Mahasudarshan are excellent for clearing toxins through their bitter taste. Sudarshan contains guduchi, chiretta (King of Bitters), black pepper, liquorice and amalaki. Once its purity is assured, Sudarshan is one of the best blood cleansers, excellent for acute infections and fevers if taken at onset, as well as for allergies, acne, eczema, boils and other *Rakta dhatu* (blood)-related conditions.

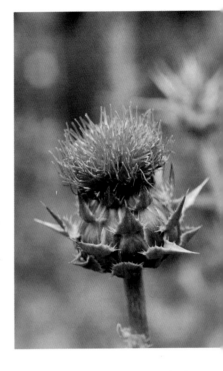

Milk thistle is one of the best remedies for the liver, helping to protect and heal it from damage caused by drugs and alcohol.

Take half a teaspoon of the powder in the morning on an empty stomach, mixed in honey as an *Anupana* or vehicle. Those who have difficulty taking such a bitter herb in this form can take Sudarshan or Mahasudarshan tablets or capsules instead.

For optimum detoxification it is important to be aware of clearing toxins through all the pathways of elimination. The bitter herbs listed above help to clear toxins through the liver. Cooling and cleansing herbs such as sariva, red sandalwood, vetiver, neem leaf, fennel, turmeric, fenugreek, cumin and manjishta can be taken regularly as teas to help clear toxins through the sweat glands and the skin. Teas made from herbs and spices (including coriander, cumin and fennel) enhance elimination through the urinary tract, while others promote elimination through the bowels, and massage and exercise help to improve circulation of the blood and lymph.

Bowel cleansers

Clearing out toxins via the bowels enhances digestion, immunity,

energy and positivity. Constipation or irregular bowel movements cause wastes to be reabsorbed into the body, creating toxins in the *Rasa dhatu* (plasma), the *Rakta dhatu* (blood), and from there the other *dhatus* (tissues). A regular bowel movement is vital for proper daily detoxification.

If the stool is very dry or slow, try adding more oil or ghee to your diet, and drink plenty of fluid, including warm water and herbal teas such as liquorice, fennel and dandelion coffee. Add spices such as turmeric, ginger, cumin and coriander to your food to enhance digestion and liver function. Eat foods with plenty of fibre, such as oats, leafy greens, and cooked or soaked prunes and figs. Avoid a *Vata*-aggravating diet and drying foods such as crackers, dried cereal and raw foods.

Gentle purgatives can be used for constipation or irregular bowel habits, especially if the stools sink rather than float, as this indicates the presence of *Ama*. Herbal purgatives cleanse the small and large intestine and can be taken on the first day of a fast, and again once every three to seven days of the fast, if there is still evidence of *Ama* in the form of a coating on the tongue. Purgative and laxative herbs are contraindicated in diarrhoea, debility or underweight, even if the tongue is coated or there are other signs of *Ama*. There are other herbs and formulae that can cleanse the bowel without being laxative.

Bitter purgatives such as rhubarb, castor oil and aloe are recommended along with warming spices such as ginger to protect the digestive fire and to burn up *Ama*.

Soothing bulk laxatives, like flaxseed and psyllium, are not recommended in *Ama* conditions as they can further clog up the system.

By far the best Ayurvedic formula for cleansing the bowel is Triphala, which is a mixture of amalaki, haritaki and bibhitaki. It not only clears *Ama*, but also raises digestive fire, improves metabolism and nourishes the deeper tissues. It is ideal for all *doshas*. Take half a teaspoon in hot water half an hour before sleep.

Aloe-vera gel is another excellent bowel cleanser and is best taken along with warming spices like ginger, black pepper

---

REMEDIES FOR CLEARING TOXINS ACCORDING TO THE *DOSHAS*:

- **For *Vata*:** Haritaki, Hingwashtaka, Lavanbhaskar
- **For *Pitta*:** Guduchi and ginger, coriander, amalaki
- **For *Kapha*:** Triphala Guggulu, Trikatu

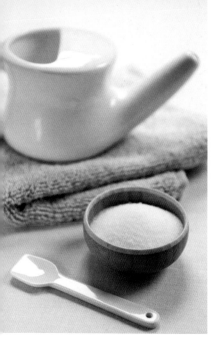

Using salt water daily in a Neti *pot will help to protect you from respiratory infections.*

Enemas (*Basti*)

Enemas are an excellent way to cleanse the colon effectively and are particularly suited to those with a *Vata* constitution. They are one of the easiest ways to flush out the colon and restore regular peristaltic movement (see Chapter 17). As Hippocrates said, 'Enema is better than any purgative/laxative medicine.'

Nasal irrigation (*Jalaneti*)

Using salt water in a *Neti* pot every day is excellent for preventing respiratory infections and treating chronic sinusitis and allergies such as hay fever and asthma.

Using the *Neti* pot, pour water at room temperature containing a little sea salt into one nostril and let it exit through the other nostril, taking care not to put your head back so that the water goes down

and turmeric. It is soothing, immune-enhancing and combats dysbiosis (pathogenic micro-organisms in the gut). It is particularly good for *Sama Pitta* and *Sama Kapha*. Take 25 ml twice daily.

Neem, garlic, ginger, guggulu, Triphala, andrographis and turmeric are excellent for combating dysbiosis. Dill, cinnamon, guduchi, fennel, amalaki and tulsi act similarly.

your throat. Any residual water can be cleared by some short, sharp breaths using the diaphragm, known as *Kapalabhati*.

Tooth and gum health

It is important to take measures to prevent tooth and gum disease, as they cause toxins from the mouth to be absorbed directly into the bloodstream. Gingivitis and pyorrhoea can cause spongy, bleeding, infected and receding gums and tooth decay. By adding antimicrobial herbs into your daily routine you can help to deter infection. Neem is a powerful antimicrobial herb, which is excellent for oral health, and can effectively combat cavity-causing bacteria and prevent bleeding gums and the build-up of tartar and plaque; use a 10 per cent neem oil to massage the gums. Clove oil is an excellent antiseptic pain-reliever, often used by dentists to numb the gums prior to giving injections. Massage the gums with a mixture of eucalyptus, clove and spearmint essential oils with sesame oil (two drops of essential oil per 5 ml of sesame oil) to prevent the build-up of bacteria in the mouth. Ginger tea is an excellent antimicrobial wash for the teeth, while diluted lemon juice makes a good whitener.

Tongue-cleaning

The surface of the tongue is a breeding ground for bacteria that can cause infection in the teeth and gums and are often responsible for bad breath. Cleaning your tongue every day after brushing your teeth is part of a traditional Ayurvedic and yogic practice, and can reduce bad breath and bacteria by up to 75 per cent. The best tongue-cleaners are made of copper.

3 Post-detoxification

The third step, or post-detoxification, is important because this is the optimum time to take *Rasayanas* – the Ayurvedic elixirs that rejuvenate the body

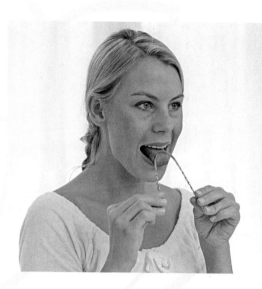

Tongue-cleansing can reduce bad breath and bacteria by up to 75 per cent.

and help stop ageing (see Chapter 18) – such as ashwagandha and Chayawanprash. With the toxins cleared out of the tissues and *srotas*, the body can better utilize the benefits of *Rasayanas*.

After spending 15–30 days preparing for cleansing and three to four weeks doing the detox, you should feel much lighter, more energetic, brighter and happier. You may well lose weight (normally 3–6 kg/7–14 lb).

Gradually return to eating more, but not necessarily to the same diet you had prior to detoxing, if this was a generally *Ama*-increasing diet. There may be a few changes that you would like to incorporate permanently into your diet. Make sure you get plenty of rest for a few days after your detox, and follow your normal Ayurvedic routine and recommended diet for your *dosha* type or *Prakruti*.

Chapter 12: Treatment of the *doshas*

The right balance of the *doshas* is fundamental to our well-being because the *doshas* influence every aspect of our lives, not only determining our physical shape and attributes, but also governing every physiological and psychological aspect of our being. In order to maintain health, or treat derangements of the *doshas* when they arise, we first have to make an assessment of the balance or imbalance of our *doshas*.

If we are out of balance, it means that our *doshas* have changed from the basic constitution that we are born with (*Prakruti*) to our present *doshic* imbalance (*Vikruti*). Rebalancing the *doshas* through the right diet, lifestyle and herbs is central to preventative health because any disturbance of the *doshas* will eventually lead to ill health, and is fundamental to the treatment of disease.

Balance of the doshas *is essential to our well-being.*

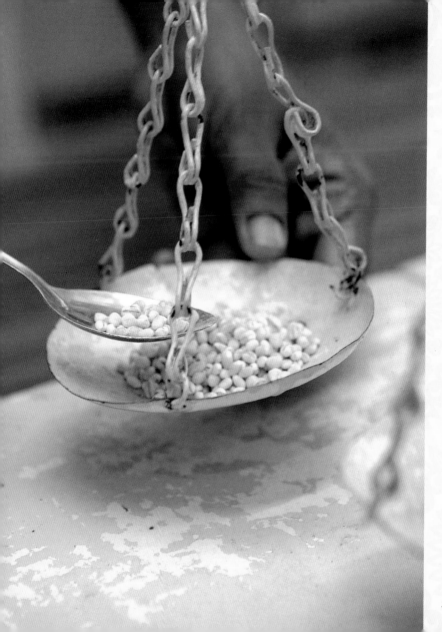

Balancing the *doshas*

Once our *Prakruti* and *Vikruti* have been established, through the various diagnostic methods incorporated into case history-taking, treatment aimed at balancing the *doshas* can begin. The aim is not to balance the *doshas per se*, but to return to the balance of our *Prakruti*.

Generally speaking, if one *dosha* is out of balance, treatment should be relatively straightforward. If two *doshas* are out of balance, it is more challenging. When all three *doshas* are out of balance, it can mean that treatment might be more palliative than curative.

When more than one *dosha* is disturbed, treatment is aimed at balancing the *dosha* that is causing the most significant symptoms. However, it is important to recognize the role of *Vata* in the development of symptoms. *Vata* is the mover and changes easily; without *Vata* the other two *doshas* cannot move into imbalance. For this reason it is always important to consider redressing the balance of *Vata* in your choice of foods and herbs, even in a *Pitta* or *Kapha* problem.

There is a variety of different ways to remedy imbalances of the *doshas*, all of which involve enhancing our relationship with the world around us. Ayurveda uses herbal medicines and wholesome foods, and addresses every aspect of daily living. The herbs, diet and lifestyle advocated for each individual patient will vary according to their effect on the three *doshas* and the individual's *Vikruti*.

> ## THE *DOSHA* QUALITIES
>
> - *Vata*: cold, light, dry, subtle, mobile, sharp, hard, rough, clear
> - *Pitta*: hot, a little wet, light, subtle, flowing, mobile, sharp, soft, smooth, clear
> - *Kapha*: cold, wet, heavy, gross, dense, static, dull, soft, smooth, cloudy

Qualities (*gunas*)

The choice of food and herbal remedy depends on its 'quality' or 'energy', which Ayurveda determines according to 20 attributes (see page 76), such as hot, cold, wet, dry, heavy or light, and these arise from the three *gunas*. In the herbal section (see Chapter 15) you will find the quality of each herb described, which will be helpful when making your choice of herbs for balancing the *doshas*. You need to use herbs with the opposite quality to that of the *dosha* that is imbalanced. So, in the case of excess *Kapha*, which is cold and damp, you need herbs that are warm and dry.

Taste

Your choice of diet and herbs to rebalance the *doshas* can be guided by their taste (see page 129). Understanding the effects on mind and body of each taste, and how this relates to the balance of the *doshas*, means that food and herbs chosen can be more specifically related to the needs of each individual person, making them more effective tools for the prevention and treatment of imbalance and disease. Generally speaking, tastes relate to the *doshas* in the following ways:

- Sweet, sour and salty substances increase *Kapha* and decrease *Vata*.

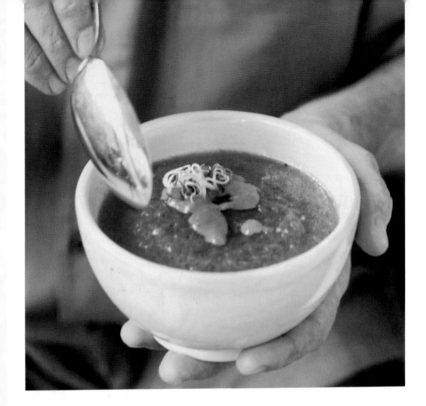

Red lentils have an astringent taste which increases Vata and reduces Pitta and Kapha.

- Sweet, bitter and astringent tastes decrease *Pitta*.
- Pungent, bitter and astringent tastes decrease *Kapha* and increase *Vata*.
- Pungent, sour and salty tastes increase *Pitta*.

Development of signs and symptoms

To understand the development of symptoms caused by a derangement of the *doshas* it is helpful to know the main sites where each *dosha* resides (see Chapter 2) and to return to the discussion of the five subtypes of the *doshas* (see page 54). The symptoms that develop begin in the main site of the *dosha* and, as they spread, they manifest mainly in the other sites related to the particular *dosha* that is involved.

The main site of *Vata* is *Apana Vata*, located in the lower abdomen and colon, which is responsible for all downward-moving impulses of elimination, including defecation, urination, menstruation, childbirth, ejaculation and the passing of wind. When *Apana Vata* is disturbed it affects these downward movements, and initially causes bowel disturbances such as wind, constipation, diarrhoea and irritable bowel syndrome. It also governs absorption of water in the large intestine and enables us to take in the full nourishment from the digestion of food, the final stage of which occurs in the large intestine. Since *Apana Vata* supports and controls all other forms of *Vata*, when it becomes disturbed it

forms the basis of most *Vata* disorders. So treatment of *Apana Vata* is the first consideration in the treatment of all *Vata* problems and this will allow the other *Vatas* to return to normal functioning.

Balancing the *Vatas*

Vata disorders are the fundamental basis of most diseases and always accompany those of *Pitta* and *Kapha*. For this reason it is always important to consider *Apana Vata* in the treatment of any disease related to all three *doshas*. Keeping all five *Vatas* in balance and properly functioning is the vital key to maintaining health. Should treatment of *Apana Vata* be overlooked, symptoms will then spread according to the six stages of disease (see page 162) and manifest in another site of *Vata*, such as in the head, mind or chest (*Prana Vata*), the throat (*Udana Vata*), the stomach and small intestine (*Samana Vata*) or the circulation (*Vyana Vata*).

Treatment of *Vata*

Vata people are changeable and forgetful. They can be very enthusiastic at the start of treatment, but easily forget to follow their diet and take their herbs, so it is important not to overwhelm them at the start of treatment and to review the situation frequently.

In order to keep *Vata* in balance, or to calm it when it is out of balance, it is helpful to understand what actually deranges *Vata*.

THE MAIN SITES
OF *VATA*

- Lower abdomen, including large bowel and genito-urinary tract
- Hips and thighs
- Bones and joints
- Nerve tissue, mind
- Ears
- Skin

Causes of *Vata* aggravation

- Irregular, erratic lifestyle, irregular eating patterns, missing meals
- Stress, grief, anxiety, fear, shock, loneliness
- Change, such as moving house/school/work/relationship/climate/country
- Flying, travelling, changing time zones, foods, etc.
- Change of season, especially autumn
- Dawn and dusk, 2–6 a.m. and 2–6 p.m.
- Too much movement, exercise, running, jumping, etc.

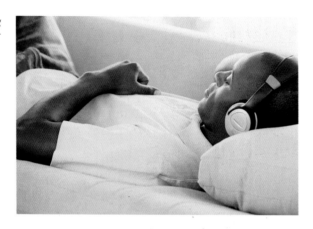

Listening to soothing music can help Vata-type anxiety.

- Suppression of natural urges, such as eating, urination, bowel movements, passing wind, resting when tired, sleeping, etc.
- Exposure to cold, dry, windy weather
- Being over the age of 50
- Lack of sleep, exhaustion
- Excess bitter, pungent and astringent foods
- Excess dry, light, rough, cold foods
- Talking too much
- Loud noise, overstimulation, doing too much, pushing yourself beyond your resources

Signs of *Vata* aggravation

- Constipation, wind, colic, distension, explosive diarrhoea (aggravated by anxiety)
- Aching pain in the bones, cracking joints, arthritis, low backache
- Fatigue, lowered resistance to infection, loss of weight
- Tinnitus, tingling and numbness
- Feeling cold, poor circulation
- Dry skin and hair, brittle nails
- Pain (cutting or migrating), poor coordination, insomnia, restless sleep, tension and anxiety,

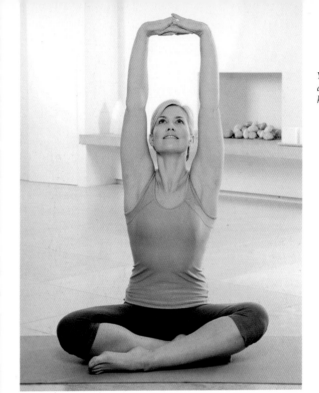

Yoga, Pranayama *and meditation all help reduce* Vata.

insecurity, mental agitation, depression, restlessness
- Neurological problems, tremors, disorientation and dizziness
  Symptoms are worse at dawn or dusk, 2–6 a.m. and 2–6 p.m. They are aggravated by cold and windy weather, and feel better in warm weather.

Treatment of *Vata* problems (*Vata Shamana*)
- Plenty of relaxation, rest and sleep; avoid overstimulation and doing too much
- Methods to reduce anxiety, including yoga, *Pranayama* (breathing exercises) and walking meditation

Ashwagandha is one of the most important herbs for balancing Vata *and is famous as a rejuvenative and adaptogen.*

- A regular routine, eating meals, and taking gentle exercise regularly
- Massage and internal and external use of oils, particularly sesame oil (see page 246), followed by the application of heat or a warm bath or shower. Oils used externally include nilyadi, sesame, narayan, mahanaryan and castor oil; ghee in food
- Light purgation using Triphala
- Nasal administration of oil (*Nasya*), often for psychological problems, such as mahanaryan oil
- *Shirodhara* (medicated water or milk or herbal oils are poured continuously on the forehead for 30–45 minutes)
- A light diet of warm, soft foods, avoiding hard, raw, dry and indigestible foods
- Mild spices such as fresh ginger, cumin, cardamom, fennel, coriander

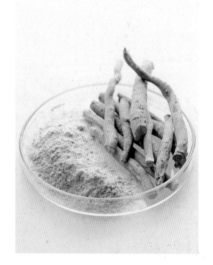

- Increasing sweet, sour and salty foods and minimizing pungent, bitter and astringent foods

Herbs

- Particularly aimed at balancing *Apana Vata*: ashwagandha, shatavari, asafoetida, brahmi, bala, gokshura, guduchi, dill, celery seed, ginger, long pepper, haritaki, guggulu, liquorice, saffron, tulsi, valerian,

VATA-REDUCING DIET

	DECREASE	INCREASE
FRUITS	Dried fruits, raw fruits, persimmons, watermelon, raw apples, pears, pomegranates, cranberries	Sweet fruits, avocados, berries, citrus fruits, plums, melons (sweet), dates (fresh), papaya, apricots, bananas (ripe), cherries, figs (fresh), grapes, mangos, peaches, prunes (soaked), pineapples
VEGETABLES	Raw vegetables, sprouts, cauliflower, potatoes, tomatoes, celery, aubergine, onions (raw), bitter melon, broccoli, salad, Brussels sprouts, spinach, peppers, kohlrabi, mushrooms, parsley, cabbage (raw)	Cooked vegetables, beets, cucumber, courgettes, leafy greens, green beans, onions (cooked), radishes, butternut squash, peas (cooked), asparagus, carrots, garlic, fennel, okra (cooked), sweet potatoes, leeks, parsnips, pumpkin
GRAINS	Bread with yeast, buckwheat, millet, rice (brown), corn, oats (dry), rye, muesli, dry crackers	Barley, rice (white and basmati), wheat, oats (cooked), amaranth, quinoa
ANIMAL FOODS	Lamb, rabbit, pork, venison	Beef, eggs, salmon, white fish, chicken, duck, turkey, seafood, sardines, tuna

VATA-REDUCING DIET

	GENERAL ADVICE
LEGUMES	No legumes except mung beans, tofu, urad dhal, red lentils
NUTS	All nuts in moderation, especially when ground
SEEDS	All seeds in moderation, especially when ground
SWEETENERS	All sweeteners except white sugar
CONDIMENTS	All spices are good, except the hot ones like chilli, dried ginger, horseradish
DAIRY FOODS	All dairy products in moderation, except cheese
OILS	All oils are good, particularly sesame, olive and ghee

cardamom, cinnamon, fenugreek, garlic, coriander, cumin, nutmeg, turmeric, frankincense, clove
• Formulae: Triphala Guggulu, Hingwashtaka, Talisadi, Trikatu, Trikulu
• *Rasayanas* (tonics): ashwagandha, shatavari, bala, gotu kola, gokshura, bacopa, kapikachu, vidari khanda, Chayawanprash as a general tonic; *Rasayana* for digestion: Trikatu

Teas
• Herbs can be taken singly as teas or made into mixtures of your choice: fresh ginger, cardamom, tulsi, clove, fennel, lemongrass, oat straw, peppermint, cinnamon

Vehicles for medicines (*Anupana*)
• Warm milk, hot water, ghee. Medicines are best taken before a meal.

Treatment of *Pitta*

Pitta types are perfectionists; once they decide to commit to getting well, they have the discipline to adhere to a diet and take their medicine on time! They are likely to have list of foods they can or cannot eat and the right containers for their herbs. For this reason it is easy for them to get the best out of treatment.

In order to keep *Pitta* in balance, or to calm it when it is out of balance, it is helpful to understand what deranges *Pitta*.

THE MAIN SITES OF *PITTA*

- Stomach and small intestine
- Liver and gall bladder
- Blood
- Skin and sweat, sebaceous glands
- Heart and mind
- Eyes

Causes of *Pitta* aggravation

- Hot weather, getting overheated
- Bright light, hot sun
- Late spring and summer
- Inflammatory situations, anger, jealousy, arguments, irritation, frustration
- Perfectionism, overambition
- Midday and midnight, 10p.m.–2 a.m. and 10a.m.–2 p.m.
- Missing meals
- Suppression of emotions
- Age 18–50
- Overwork, overcommitment, overcompetitive environment
- Pungent, sour and salty foods, fried foods

- Caffeine, hot spices, alcohol and drugs
- Going to bed late
- Too much reading at night

Signs of *Pitta* aggravation

- Inflammation, often starting in the stomach and intestines, causing heartburn, acidity, gastritis and peptic ulcers, appendicitis
- Inflammatory skin problems, such as eczema, urticaria, herpes and boils
- Tonsillitis, bronchitis
- Blood disorders, anaemia, high blood pressure
- Bleeding tendency, such as nosebleeds, heavy periods
- Eye problems such as conjunctivitis, styes and blepharitis (inflammation of the eyelid)
- Heat and burning symptoms, fevers, profuse sweat
- Thirst, increased appetite, hypoglycaemia, dizziness, diarrhoea

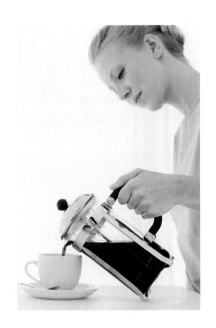

Coffee is stimulating, pungent and heating and it aggravates Pitta.

- Liver and gall-bladder problems, hepatitis
- Yellow discoloration (of the eyes, skin, nails, teeth and urine)
- Cystitis, burning urination, urinary-tract infections
- Headaches and migraine

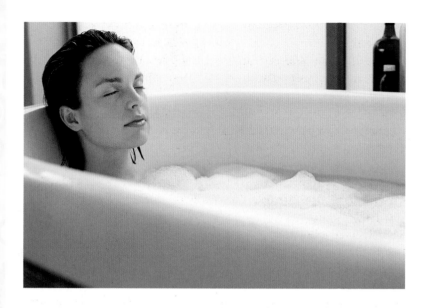

Plenty of rest, relaxation and cool baths will reduce the heat of Pitta.

- Hormonal problems, PMS
- Irritability, intolerance, anger, aggression, arrogance, perfectionism, obsessions, overcompetitiveness, anorexia, addictions, alcoholism, insomnia

    Symptoms are worse in heat and at 10p.m.–2 a.m. and 10a.m.–2 p.m. and better in cool weather.

Treatment of *Pitta* problems (*Pitta Shamana*)

- Relaxation and rest, going to bed early, 10 p.m. being ideal
- Avoiding overwork and burning the candle at both ends
- Avoiding excessive exercise, especially when it is hot
- Avoiding inflammatory situations, stressful people and situations

- Drinking plenty of cool water, aloe-vera juice
- Relaxing in cool areas, such as by water, swimming, walking by the sea
- When hot, taking cool baths with cooling herbs or essential oils, including chamomile, lavender, sandalwood, geranium, jasmine, lemongrass or rose
- *Pranayama* such as alternate nostril breathing
- Gentle laxatives such as dandelion root or Triphala to reduce excess *Pachaka Pitta*

- Massage oils with coconut or sunflower oil, aloe vera, bringaraj, nilyadi or brahmi oil
- Counselling, talking, meditation to release suppressed emotions/anger
- Soft words/music, uncompetitive activities
- Plenty of sweet, bitter and astringent foods and herbs
- Reduction of pungent, spicy, fried, sour and salty foods
- Avoiding alcohol, tobacco and recreational drugs

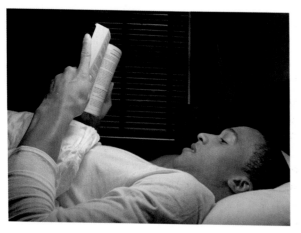

Reading books late into the night can aggravate Pitta.

PITTA-REDUCING DIET

	DECREASE	INCREASE
FRUITS	Sour fruits, berries, cherries, grapefruit, lemons, plums (sour), peaches, persimmons, apricots, bananas, cranberries, grapes (green), oranges (sour), papaya, pineapples (sour)	Sweet fruits, avocados, figs, mangos, oranges (sweet), pineapples (sweet), pomegranates, raisins, apples, grapes (dark), melons, pears, plums (sweet), prunes
VEGETABLES	Pungent vegetables, carrots, garlic, peppers (hot), spinach, beets, aubergines, raw onions and garlic, radishes, tomatoes	Sweet or bitter vegetables, broccoli, cabbage, cauliflower, green beans, lettuce, okra, parsley, potatoes, courgettes, asparagus, Brussels sprouts, cucumber, celery, leafy greens, mushrooms, peas, peppers (green), sprouts
GRAINS	Buckwheat, millet, rice (brown), corn, oats (dry), rye	Barley, rice (basmati), wheat, oats (cooked), rice (white)
ANIMAL FOODS	Beef, lamb, seafood, eggs (yolk), pork	Chicken or turkey (white meat), rabbit, venison, eggs (white), prawns (small amount), white fish
DAIRY FOODS	Buttermilk, sour cream, cheese, yoghurt	Butter (unsalted), ghee, cottage cheese, milk
OILS	Almond, safflower, corn, sesame	Coconut, sunflower, olive, soy

PITTA-REDUCING DIET

	GENERAL ADVICE
LEGUMES	All legumes except lentils
NUTS	No nuts except coconut
SEEDS	No seeds except sunflower and pumpkin
SWEETENERS	All sweeteners except molasses and honey
CONDIMENTS	No spices except coriander, cinnamon, cardamom, fennel, fresh ginger, turmeric, long pepper and a little black pepper

Herbs

- Coriander, cumin, rose, bacopa, gotu kola, bringaraj, sariva, gokshura, aloe vera, amalaki, turmeric, shatavari, guduchi, punarnava, manjishta, neem, liquorice, saffron
- Formulae: Mahasudarshan, Pippaliamla (pippali and amla), Nimbadi (neem and guduchi), Pushyanuga (a combination of many herbs), Panchatikta ghrita
- *Rasayanas*: amalaki, rose, sariva, shatavari, bringaraj, aloe vera juice, guduchi; *Rasayana* for the brain: bacopa, gotu kola and ghee

Teas

- Drink plenty of teas, lukewarm to cool
- Chamomile, hibiscus, liquorice, cumin, coriander, fennel, rose, brahmi, mint, lemongrass
- Dandelion coffee

Vehicles for medicine (*Anupana*)

- Aloe-vera juice, ghee, cool water. Medicines prepared in ghee are good nerve tonics for *Pitta*. Ghee combines well with bitter herbs, enhancing them by its *Pitta*-reducing properties. They are usually followed by milk.

Treatment of *Kapha*

Kapha types are generally strong and resilient and do not tend to get ill often. When they do, symptoms are likely to be mild and non-serious. They are likely not to seek treatment until the symptoms have progressed somewhat. Once they start treatment they will stick at it, but symptoms will be slow to change.

In order to keep *Kapha* balanced, or to calm it when it is out of balance, it is helpful to understand what actually increases *Kapha* in the first place.

THE MAIN SITES OF *KAPHA*

- Stomach, mouth, tongue
- Respiratory system, throat, mucous membranes
- Head
- Pancreas
- Lymph
- Fat

Causes of *Kapha* aggravation

- Sleeping in the daytime, excessive sleep, getting up late
- Lack of exercise and change, laziness
- Cold, damp weather, winter
- Early morning and evening, 6–10 a.m. and 6–10 p.m.
- Not eating regularly, overeating
- Excess sweet, sour and salty foods
- Excess heavy, cold and damp foods

Signs of *Kapha* aggravation

- Colds, catarrh, coughs, bronchial congestion, hay fever, asthma

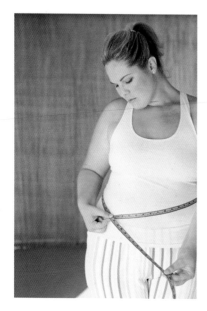

Excess Kapha *is related to slow metabolism causing weight to increase.*

- Possessiveness, acquisitiveness, greed, stubbornness, aversion to change, blocking out emotions
- Low thyroid function, high cholesterol

  Symptoms are worse in cold, damp weather and at 6–10 a.m. and 6–10 p.m.

Treatment of *Kapha* problems (*Kapha Shamana*)

- More exercise, vigorous activity, doing different things, trying to be open-minded
- Reduction of sleep if excessive, getting up well before 8 a.m. (6 a.m. is preferable!)
- Inhalation of oil/steam, application of heat
- Avoiding sweet, sour and salty foods
- Increasing pungent, bitter and astringent foods

- Low *Agni* (digestive fire), slow digestion and metabolism, excess salivation, nausea and heaviness after eating, constipation
- Overweight, obesity, metabolic syndrome, Type 2 diabetes
- Fluid retention, lymphatic congestion
- Lethargy, laziness, poor motivation, foggy-mindedness
- Poor circulation

KAPHA-REDUCING DIET

	DECREASE	INCREASE
FRUITS	Sweet and sour fruits, bananas, figs (fresh), grapes, melons, pineapples, avocados, grapefruit, lemons, oranges, papaya, plums	Apples, berries, cranberries, mangoes, pears, pomegranates, raisins, apricots, cherries, figs (dry), peaches, persimmons, prunes
VEGETABLES	Sweet and juicy vegetables, sweet potatoes, courgettes, cucumber, tomatoes	Pungent bitter vegetables, beets, Brussels sprouts, carrots, celery, garlic, lettuce, okra, parsley, peppers, radishes, sprouts, broccoli, cabbage, cauliflower, aubergines, leafy greens, mushrooms, onions, peas, potatoes (white), spinach
GRAINS	Buckwheat, millet, rice (brown), corn, oats (dry), rye	Barley, rice (basmati), wheat, oats (cooked), rice (white)
ANIMAL FOODS	Beef, pork, lamb, seafood	Chicken or turkey (dark meat), rabbit, venison, prawns

	GENERAL ADVICE
LEGUMES	All legumes except kidney beans, soy beans, black lentils and mung beans
NUTS	No nuts at all
SEEDS	No seeds except sunflower and pumpkin
SWEETENERS	No sweeteners except raw honey
CONDIMENTS	All spices are good except salt
DAIRY FOODS	No dairy products except ghee and goat milk
OILS	No oils except almond, corn or sunflower in small amounts

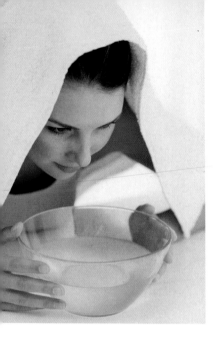

Inhalations of stimulating and decongesting herbs can be used to clear excess Kapha.

cinnamon, cloves, black pepper, fennel, aloe vera juice, cardamom, guduchi, gurmar, guggulu, kanchanara
- Formulae: Trikatu, Triphala, Triphala Guggulu, Talisadi with lime juice
- *Rasayanas*: for digestion: Trikatu, Hingwashtaka; for thyroid problems: Kanchanar Guggulu, Triphala Guggulu

Teas
- Ginger, hot water and lime juice, celery seed, cinnamon, tulsi, cardamom, chai, peppermint, fennel, thyme, cumin

Vehicles for medicines (*Anupana*)
- Honey, hot water. Medicines are best taken after a meal.
- Oils for *nasya* or inhalation.

- Eating a light diet with hot foods and regular meals
- Drinking plenty of warming drinks
- Adding hot spices to cooking
- Nasal administration of oils (*Nasya*), including eucalyptus, nilyadi and vacha oils

Herbs
- Punarnava, turmeric, ginger, pippali, fenugreek, asafoetida, cayenne, tulsi, bibhitaki, haritaki,

245

Warm-oil massage (*Abhyanga*)

Using oils internally and externally (*Snehana*) is important in Ayurveda, particularly as a prelude to detoxification. Applying warm sesame oil to the body is relaxing and rejuvenating; it increases energy flow, improves digestion and helps the release of stress, pent-up emotions and toxins.

Massage with oil has a significant detoxifying effect. By stimulating the tissues under the skin, it helps prevent toxins from accumulating in the system and helps them drain to the gut for elimination. It is rejuvenation and detoxification in one completely blissful experience!

Preparing the oil

For external use, sesame oil is prepared by heating the oil in a *bain marie* (double boiler) with one or two drops of water until the water evaporates. Heating the oil has been shown to increase the antioxidant effect. When taken internally, cold-pressed sesame oil is used to moisten dry *Vata* membranes and tissues and to soften and loosen dry and hardened toxins. It is best taken raw, at a dose of one to two tablespoons daily.

> **CAUTION**
>
> **Avoid *Abhyanga* immediately after administering enemas, emetics or purgatives, during the first stages of fever or if suffering from indigestion.**

OILS FOR THE *DOSHAS*

- **Oils for *Vata*:** Sesame, almond, castor, mahanaryan, ashwagandha, bala
- **Oils for *Pitta*:** Coconut, olive, sunflower, brahmi, bringaraj; ghee for internal use
- **Oils for *Kapha*:** Vacha, mustard, flaxseed

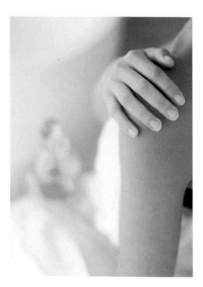

Massage the oil into the skin and leave for 5 to 15 minutes before taking a hot bath or shower.

How to perform *Abhyanga*

Daily *Abhyanga* is best done in the morning. Rub the oil all over the body and leave it to soak in for five to fifteen minutes, before taking a warm bath or shower. This allows time for the oil to be absorbed and nourish and detoxify the tissue layers. The warm bath or shower opens the pores, allowing the oil to permeate further into the body.

To ease tension and relieve insomnia, it is best to apply the oil in the evening before bed, and this should include oiling the soles of the feet. The oil should be at room temperature in the summer, but

The rich oil expressed from sesame seeds is packed with antioxidants.

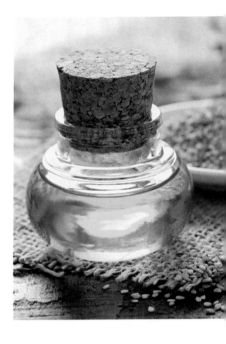

needs to be warmed in the winter. Herbal or essential oils can be added to enhance specific desired effects, such as lavender oil for stress and tension, frankincense for arthritic pain, or ginger to increase the circulation.

The therapeutic value of sesame oil

Sesame oil is one of the most important tools of Ayurvedic medicine. It is one of the best remedies for balancing *Vata* and, because *Vata* derangement lies behind imbalances of the other two *doshas*, deserves pride of place as a remedy. The rich, almost odourless oil expressed from sesame seeds is stable and contains antioxidants that stop it from going rancid (if properly stored), and thus make it popular as cooking oil in India and China. It is highly nutritious, rich in vitamins A, B and E, as well as the minerals iron, calcium, magnesium, copper, silicic acid and phosphorus. It contains antioxidants, linoleic acid and alpha-linoleic acid, as well as lecithin, and this may help to explain its benefits to the brain and nervous system. Like olive oil, sesame oil is considered good for lowering harmful cholesterol levels. White seeds produce the most oil, but in India they say the best oil for healing is extracted from black sesame seeds.

In India the use of sesame oil in *Abhyanga* is part of everyday life and an important aspect of Ayurveda. It is the favourite oil for massage as its chemical structure gives it a unique ability to penetrate the skin, nourishing and detoxifying even the deepest tissue layers. It is said to benefit all seven tissues (*dhatus*). It is the best oil for balancing *Vata*, but can also be used sparingly for *Pitta* and *Kapha*.

Used regularly, sesame oil is wonderful for reducing stress and tension, nourishing the nervous system and preventing nervous disorders, relieving fatigue and insomnia, and promoting strength and vitality. Those patients who use it daily have reported feeling stronger, more resilient to stress, with increased energy and better resistance to infection. Its rejuvenating properties ease pain and muscle spasm, such as sciatica, period pain, colic, backache and joint pain. The antioxidants explain its reputation for slowing the ageing process and increasing longevity – certainly regular oiling of the skin restores moisture to the skin, keeping it soft, flexible and young-looking. It also lubricates the body internally, particularly the joints and bowels, and eases symptoms of dryness, such as irritating coughs, cracking joints and hard stools.

Research into the healing effect of applying sesame oil is beginning to emerge. Those who practise it daily have found they have less bacterial infection on their skin and that it eases joint problems. This may be related to the linoleic acid that makes up 40 per cent of sesame oil and has antibacterial and anti-inflammatory effects. It stimulates antibody production and enhances immunity. It also has anti-cancer properties and has been shown to inhibit the growth of malignant melanoma.

Chapter 13: **Treatment of the *dhatus***

When the seven *dhatus* (tissues) are functioning at their best, they are described as being *Dhatu-sara*, meaning functioning optimally, and the result is vibrant health.

Dhatu-sara qualities

- **Plasma (*Rasa-sara*)**: good complexion, glowing skin, smooth, shiny hair, good stamina, joyful resilient disposition

- **Blood (*Rakta-sara*)**: good circulation with warm hands and feet, red lips and conjunctiva, rosy cheeks, pink tongue, warm skin, good energy, happy disposition

- **Muscle (*Mamsa-sara*)**: well-developed and toned muscles, good stamina, courage, stability, beautiful developed body shape

- **Fat (*Meda-sara*)**: good covering of fat and lubrication of the joints, stools, hair, eyes, etc., lustrous hair, melodious voice, emotionally strong, full of love, joy and compassion

- **Bone (*Asthi-sara*)**: strong bones and teeth, tall frame, thick hair and nails, big joints, patient, stable, with good endurance

- **Nerve (*Majja-sara*)**: big, clear eyes, sharp mind, sensitive, good memory, resilient to pain

- **Reproductive organs (*Shukra-sara*)**: lustrous eyes, well-formed sexual organs, able to love.

When the dhatus *are at the their best our skin glows, our hair is lustrous, our mind sharp.*

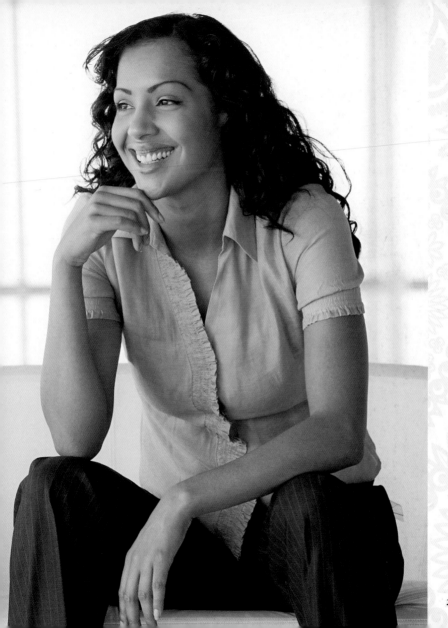

How the *doshas* affect the *dhatus*

While disturbances of the *doshas* lie behind the physiological and psychological changes that occur in mind and body, the *dhatus* are the actual sites of disease. When they are adversely affected by problems in the *srotas* (channels), they become known as *dushya*, meaning 'that which can be spoiled'.

When a *dosha* increases and enters into the respective *dhatus*, it creates disorders, particularly if there is an inherent weakness in that *dhatu*. This can be due to trauma or past injury/*Karma* (action) and so it can be inherited. The *dosha* enters with the *Agni* (digestive fire) first into the *Rasa dhatu* (plasma tissue), then into *Rakta* (blood tissue), and so on through the seven *dhatus* until it reaches *Ojas* (energy and immunity). However, in some circumstances where *Ojas* is depleted, *Vata* can become retrograde (*Ojas, Shukra, Majja*, etc.), which is more difficult to cure.

Entry of *Vata* into the *dhatus*

- ***Rasa***: Dehydration, numbness, poor circulation, dry, cold or cracked skin, goose pimples, scleroderma (contraction of the skin), eczema, psoriasis, dry cough, itching from dryness, lack of sweating, pricking pains.
  Useful herbs: Fresh ginger, tulsi, shatavari

- ***Rakta***: Gout, heart disease, hypertension, blood clots, varicose veins, arteriosclerosis, easy bruising, palpitations, poor circulation, cold extremities, slow-healing wounds, anaemia

Useful herbs: Amalaki, shatavari, liquorice, gotu kola

- *Mamsa*: Bell's palsy, paralysis, myomas (uterine fibroids), weakness and wasting of the muscles, cramps, twitches, tics, tiredness, lack of flexibility, muscle pain, tremors, poor coordination. **Useful herbs**: Ashwagandha, bala, ghee, kapikachu

- *Medas*: Diabetes, tuberculosis, lipoma (tumour of the fatty tissue), drying of the fat tissue, loss of weight, wasting, lack of sweating, sunken eyes, prominent bones, hard and small lumps, loose joints, lower backache. **Useful herbs**: Liquorice, vidarikanda, shatavari, ashwagandha

- *Asthi*: Osteoporosis, sensitive teeth, brittle nails, dry hair, loss of hair, cracking joints, bone and joint pain, cavities in teeth, degenerative arthritis. **Useful**

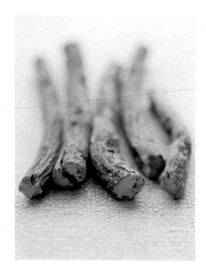

Liquorice calms Vata *and* Pitta *and can be used for entry of* Vata *into* Rakta dhatu.

herbs: Guggulu, ashwagandha, frankincense, turmeric

- *Majja*: Blurred vision, anaemia, neurological and muscular problems, multiple sclerosis, epilepsy, sciatica, numbness, neuralgia, tremors, dizziness, tinnitus, paralysis, psychological problems, fear and anxiety.

Useful herbs: Ashwagandha, jatamansi (an excellent *tridoshic* herb for the nervous system), vacha, brahmi, kapikachu

- *Shukra*: Infertility, impotence, low immunity, tuberculosis, low sperm count, prostatitis, painful or scanty periods, uterine cysts, fibroids, fear, anxiety, feeling unloved. **Useful herbs**: Ashwagandha, kapikachu, vidarikanda, bala, shatavari

- *Ojas*: Lowered immunity (repeated infections), profuse weakness. **Useful herbs**: Vidari, ashwagandha, shatavari, amalaki, bala

Entry of *Pitta* into the *dhatus*

- *Rasa*: Red, inflamed skin, yellowish discoloration, high fevers, swollen lymph nodes, sore throat, rashes, acne, eczema, urticaria, easy bruising. **Useful herbs**: Neem, aloe vera, peppermint, Mahasudarshan

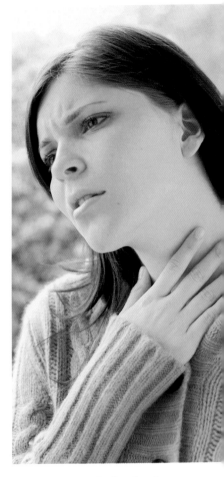

Sore throats and swollen lymph nodes are caused by entry of Pitta *into* Rasa dhatu.

- *Rakta*: Inflammatory skin problems, eczema, psoriasis, infections, boils, cholecystitis (inflammation of the gall bladder), jaundice, hepatitis, enlarged liver and spleen, anaemia, heat in the hands and feet, hot flushes, bleeding disorders. **Useful herbs**: Neem, manjishta, guduchi, amalaki

- *Mamsa*: Gastritis, enteritis, colitis, ulcers, heart problems, abscesses, gingivitis, appendicitis, fibromyalgia, infection of muscle tissue, chronic fever, bursitis. **Useful herbs**: Guduchi, Kaishore Guggulu, turmeric

- *Medas*: Boils, abscesses, tumours, diabetes, infections in fat tissue, excess sweating, excess urination, blood in urine, urinary-tract infections. **Useful herbs**: Neem, turmeric, manjishta, shankapushpi

- *Asthi*: Osteomyelitis, inflammatory arthritis, burning pain in the joints and bones, bone abscess. **Useful herbs**: Kaishore Guggulu, gotu kola

- *Majja*: Neuritis, meningitis, sciatica, numbness, headaches, anaemia. **Useful herbs**: Gotu kola, brahmi, bringaraj, jatamansi

- *Shukra*: Heavy periods, pelvic inflammatory disease, low sperm count, low fertility and immunity, drying of the reproductive fluids, painful, frequent periods, mid-cycle bleeding, swollen testicles or prostate, blood in semen, prostatitis, orchitis (swelling of the testicles), epididymitis (swelling of the epididymis). **Useful herbs**: Shankapushpi, rose, guduchi, safed musli (a body-building herb and aphrodisiac), ashoka, shatavari

- *Ojas*: Hyperpyrexia (abnormally high fever), low immunity. **Useful herbs**: Amalaki, gotu kola, guduchi, bringaraj

Entry of *Kapha* into the *dhatus*

- *Rasa*: Asthma, bronchitis, wet eczema, warts, cysts, fungal infections of the skin, pale, cold, clammy skin, cough with white sputum, swollen glands, nausea, lymphatic congestion, oedema, mild fevers, sinus congestion. **Useful herbs**: Dry ginger, kanchanara, Trikatu, pippali, turmeric

- *Rakta*: Anaemia, bile congestion, gall stones, high cholesterol, hypertension, arteriosclerosis, leucopenia (low white blood cell count), blood clots, anaemia, embolism. **Useful herbs**: Manjishta, kutki (a cooling herb), daruharidra (a liver-regulator), guggulu

- *Mamsa*: Oedema, heavy, tired and swollen muscles, heart disorders, congestive heart failure, myomas, cystic swelling on the muscle tendon, muscular hypertrophy. **Useful herbs**: Kanchanar Guggulu, arjuna, turmeric, punarnava

- *Medas*: Excess fat tissue with overweight, heaviness, tiredness, cold sweats, fibroids, lipomas, diabetes, fatty degeneration of the liver. **Useful herbs**: Kutki, Triphala Guggulu, gurmar

- *Asthi*: Bone spurs, osteoma, swollen arthritic joints, excess hair. **Useful herbs**: Punarnava Guggulu, Gokshuradi Guggulu

- *Majja*: Neurological problems, multiple sclerosis, lack of nervous sensitivity, slow responses, lethargy, depression, anaemia, brain tumours. **Useful herbs**: Brahmi, vacha, frankincense

- *Shukra*: Sexual dysfunction, infertility, uterine tumours, cysts, fibroids, benign prostatic hypertrophy, lowered immunity, benign tumours, tumours of the testicles, diabetes, prostatic

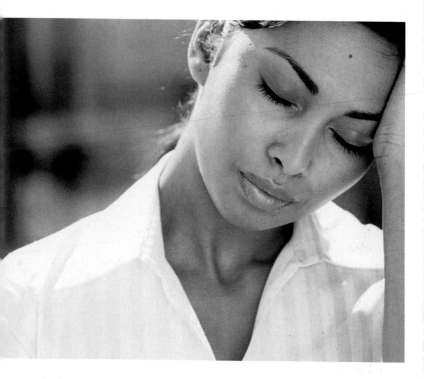

calculi (stones in the prostate). **Useful herbs**: Kapikachu, gokshura, ashwagandha

Entry of Kapha *into* Majja dhatu *can cause lethargy and depression.*

- *Ojas*: Low immunity, repeated pneumonia. **Useful herbs**: Pippali, bibhitaki, gokshura, guggulu

Chapter 14: **Ayurveda and the mind**

The mind has been called the mirror of pure awareness, which shines the light of our inner selves (the Atman) the unconditioned world beyond space and time. The mind can be experienced as awareness, intelligence and wisdom, because the light of pure awareness shines through it. The mind is the vehicle of awareness – it is not awareness itself. It reflects consciousness, which resides in the heart and pervades our whole being. If we remain in the mind we stay in the conditioned world, while liberated into pure consciousness we are free.

If we really inquire into the nature of the mind, we take a journey into our own being, becoming both the observer and the observed. We will discover all the forces working within us and will see how each of us is a microcosm of the macrocosm, a replica of the cosmos, our inner self or consciousness, one with pure passive awareness (Brahma). As the Charaka Samhita states, 'One who sees equally the entire universe in his own self and his own self in the entire universe is in possession of true knowledge.'

The mind is a mirror of pure awareness, which shines the light of our inner selves.

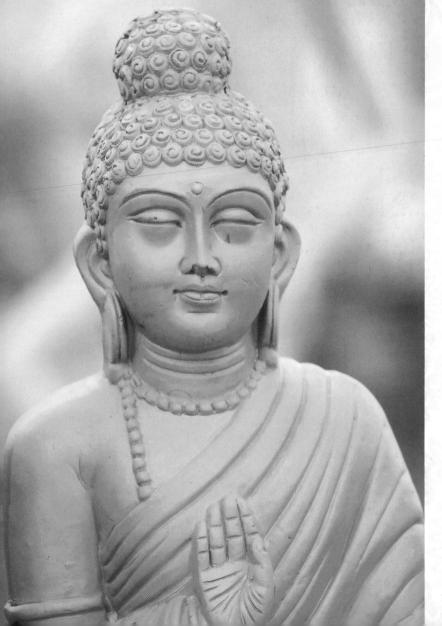

The subtle anatomy of the mind

Manovahasrotas are the subtle channels of the mind. According to the ancient texts, the channel or *srota* of the mind is the whole body, opening into the sense organs.

In this sense Ayurveda is a truly holistic system. There is no real mind-body separation, as the body is said to be the crystallization of the mind. With the help of Ayurvedic wisdom it is possible to have a broader understanding of the mind that includes our physical body and our immortal innermost self.

Mind and heart

In Ayurveda the mind and heart are one and the same. The mind is said to reside in the heart, and this means the physical heart as well as the heart of our pure awareness.

All three *doshas* reside in the heart. It is the seat of *Prana, Tejas* and *Ojas*, the subtle aspects of the *doshas* and the three *gunas Sattva, Rajas* and *Tamas*. This means that our mental and emotional state is influenced by the balance of these qualities; and likewise the mind has the power to influence our physical health. Every thought and feeling we have, every change of mood, our likes and dislikes, attractions and aversions have their impact on the *doshas* and subsequently on our health. Mental health is a state of sensory, mental, intellectual and spiritual well-being.

Universal and cosmic consciousness

According to *Sankhya* philosophy (see page 18), *Purusha* is the

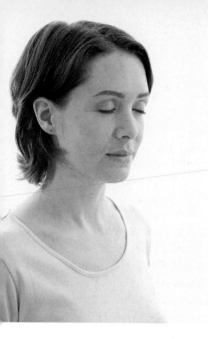

Every thought and feeling that we have has an impact on the doshas and subsequently our health.

consciousness increases in density and results in matter that produces mind, the senses and the five elements.

Mahat is the cosmic intelligence that underlies creation and all the laws and principles followed by everything in the manifest world. *Mahat* is universal and individual; it is the great truths behind life, the universal or divine mind, right down to the cellular level. Each cell has micro-*mahat*, or cellular awareness, governing its intelligence, which enables it to maintain the correct metabolic activity for its particular type.

all-pervading universal consciousness, the supreme intelligence. *Prakruti* (primordial nature) is the force of creation behind everything in the universe, both gross and subtle. It is composed of three prime qualities, or *gunas: Sattva, Rajas* and *Tamas*. The Atman is the inner self, which is divine – God within. Pure

The inner aspect of the mind

The inner aspect (*Antahkarana*) of the mind is composed of four parts:
- *Buddhi* (inner wisdom)
- *Chitta* (the storehouse of our experiences)
- *Manas* (the outer mind)
- *Ahamkara* (ego/the sense of 'I-ness').

Buddhi

In the individual soul *Mahat* becomes *Buddhi*, from the word *Buddh*, which (like the word Buddha) means 'to become awake', 'to understand' or 'to know'. It is the intelligence of the soul through which we can discern the truth, and it gives us a sense of individuality. *Buddhi* is that inner dimension of the heart/mind that is attracted to Brahma (universal consciousness), the part of us that can become enlightened once it is freed from outer attachments. It is described in the Katha Upanishad (I, 3), where it is compared to the driver of a horse and carriage: the driver's reins represent the lower mind (*Manas*), the horses are the five senses and the carriage represents the body.

Chitta

This is the storehouse of all our experiences, including *Samskaras* – the influences from all our experiences (including past lifetimes) that unconsciously govern many of our mental and emotional traits. The mind soaks up impressions taken in by the five senses and stores them in *Chitta* in the heart, which then becomes the container of thoughts, sensations and feelings. These have a direct impact on our experience of life, for they become the glasses through which we see the world, and in turn affect our mental and physical health significantly.

Chitta nadi is the channel through which our *Samskaras* flow into our outer world and colour our experience, and then the experiences from the outer world of the senses flow to the inner world of the heart, where they are stored. The outward flow gives rise to the outer mind and emotions, which is *Manas*, and the inner flow goes to the inner mind, which is *Buddhi*.

Manas

The outer aspect of *Chitta* is called *Manas* – our general thinking faculty. It is concerned with the organization of information received from the outer world of the five senses.

Since this aspect of the mind is connected to the senses, it can experience endless mental and emotional sensations, which involve worldly desires and attachment to outer form, which bring with them turbulence and suffering.

It is *Manas* that pulls consciousness to be incarnated or reincarnated into material existence as an individual soul. The wisdom and discernment of *Buddhi* takes an incarnate soul back toward the spiritual heart by releasing our identification with the material world and helping us relinquish worldly desires and thereby enabling liberation (*Moksha*).

Ahamkara

Ahamkara gives us a sense of individuality, I-ness, synonymous with our concept of the ego. It creates the illusion of 'me' and 'mine' – that we are independent individuals with our own private consciousness, rather than part of the universal or divine consciousness. Thus it creates duality and a feeling of separateness from others.

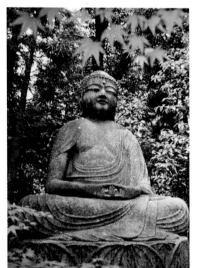

Buddhi is the intelligence of the soul and comes from the word 'Buddha' which means 'to become awake'.

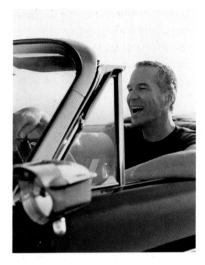

Our Ahamkara *may cause us to feel identified with our new car, imagining it to give us status.*

Ahamkara is created by *Buddhi* and so it is ultimately subordinate to it.

When our mind is in a state of *Ahamkara* we can be unconsciously identified with something that is usually outside ourselves. It could be a material thing (such as a new car), which we feel gives us some kind of status, or a concept or idea (such as a religious belief) that, if threatened, might even cause us to go to war. In *Ahamkara* a state of *Rajas* (agitation/energy) predominates because, by identifying with a small part of creation and rejecting everything else as 'not me', we become prone to mental suffering such as pride, anger, hatred and jealousy.

The wisdom of *Buddhi*

The heart provides a bridge between individual mind (*Buddhi*) and universal mind and awareness (*Mahat*). Without identification or separation of *Ahamkara*, the individual mind can experience its true nature as the universal mind. The ultimate cause of disease is ignorance, the illusion that the 'I-ness' is real; so the cure for all disease lies in the discriminative wisdom of *Buddhi*, which can dispel this illusion, and real health is liberation from the cycle of reincarnation and suffering and the realization that we are *Purusha*, or pure consciousness.

The mental forms of the *doshas*

Prana, Tejas and *Ojas* are the more subtle forms of the three *doshas*, which exert their influence in the mind. They fulfil similar functions to those of their three forms in the physical brain (*Prana Vata, Sadhaka Pitta* and *Tarpaka Kapha*), but on a more subtle level. They are also disturbed by those things that disturb the *doshas* generally (see Chapter 12).

Prana

The mental form of *Vata* is called *Prana*, and is our life force and the breath of life. At a cellular level it is the flow of intelligence, the communication between each cell that holds our organism together. *Prana* gives us inspiration and positivity, the will to live, grow and heal ourselves, and connects us with our inner self. When *Prana* is still, it becomes pure blissful awareness.

Too much *Prana* causes loss of mental control, as the life force loses its connection with the brain and body, leading to loss of sensory and motor coordination, and predisposes us to learning and behavioural problems, such as Attention Deficit Hyperactivity Disorder (ADHD). We might feel ungrounded, stressed and alienated, with a poor sense of identity.

Too little *Prana* causes lack of mental energy, enthusiasm and curiosity. Our life force and healing energy are diminished, and receptivity and creativity are inhibited. The mind and senses can be dull and heavy, we lose motivation, and our attitudes can become conservative and rigid.

Tejas

The mental form of *Pitta* is called *Tejas*; it is the fire of the mind, cellular intelligence. *Tejas* promotes intelligence, reason, passion to learn, focus, self-discipline, perception and mental clarity. One can potentially experience pure bliss. Too much *Tejas* can cause an overly critical and discriminating mind, doubt, anger, irritability and enmity. People with excess *Tejas* can be hard to please and prone to temper tantrums. Too little *Tejas* can cause an inability to enquire or discern, accepting things uncritically and losing the power to learn from experience. It can cause us to be passive and impressionable, and overly influenced by others so that we lack purpose and lose direction.

Ojas

The mental form of *Kapha* is *Ojas*, the essential vital fluid of the body in subtle form in the mind. *Ojas* promotes mental strength, stability, endurance, patience, calmness, good memory and sustained concentration, happiness, contentment and bliss. It connects and sustains our physical-mental-spiritual well-being. *Ojas* is essentially our peace of mind and is regenerated through meditation. Excess *Ojas* causes heaviness and dullness in the mind, as well as complacency and an unwillingness to change or grow.

Balancing actions

Generally high *Ojas* is much less of a problem than excess *Prana* or *Tejas*, which are the main factors in mental disorders. High *Prana* dries out *Ojas*, and high *Tejas* burns it up. Excess *Prana* and *Tejas* go along then with low *Ojas*. According to Charaka, 'when *Ojas* is low the person is fearful, weak, worries, has deranged senses, poor complexion, weak mind, is rough and thin'. We may lack self-confidence, have difficulty concentrating, poor memory and a lack of faith. Nervous exhaustion or mental problems can develop.

Prana, *Tejas* and *Ojas* control *Vata*, *Pitta* and *Kapha* in the body. Factors that balance them include meditation, prayer, self-study, deep sleep and relaxation, the right use of colours, aromas and gems. *Prana* in particular is strengthened by spending time in

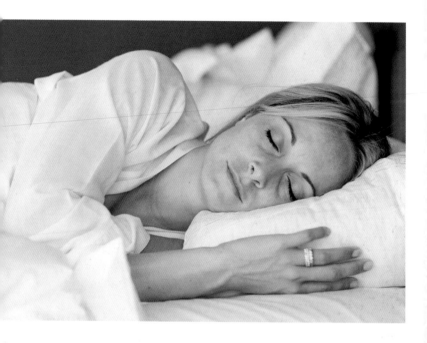

Deep sleep helps to keep Prana, Tejas *and* Ojas *in balance.*

nature and by communion with the 'cosmic forces'. Virtues such as faith, love, receptivity, compassion and understanding are also important. Factors that cause imbalances of *Prana, Tejas* and *Ojas* include the use of drugs (medical or recreational), excess exposure to mass-media influences, televisions or computers, and over-strong sensations, such as overly bright colours, loud noise, stress, excess or pretended emotions and incorrect meditation practices. Excess breathing exercises (*Pranayama*) can aggravate *Prana*.

The *doshas* and the mind

We can observe the effect that disturbance of the three *doshas* has on *Prana*, *Tejas* and *Ojas* through mental and emotional disturbances that we commonly experience. The three main subtypes of the *doshas* that relate particularly to our mental and emotional state are described below.

Prana Vata

Connected to higher cerebral functions, *Prana Vata* governs the movement of the mind, thoughts and feelings. It could be correlated with the brain's neuroelectrical activity. It promotes enthusiasm, inspiration, mental adaptability, the ability to communicate and coordinate ideas. When disturbed, it can give rise to restlessness, anxiety, insecurity, fear, insomnia, nightmares and physical neurological problems, such as palpitations, tremors, epilepsy and dementia. *Prana Vata* is considered the most important aspect of *Vata* and directs the other four sub-*doshas* of *Vata*. Since *Vata* leads the body as a whole, keeping *Prana Vata* in balance significantly affects our general health.

Sadhaka Pitta

Our mental and emotional health is very much affected by *Sadhaka Pitta* – the *Pitta* in the heart and mind. It governs the biochemical substances (neurotransmitters such as dopamine and serotonin) in the brain and is responsible for blood flow through the heart, and the emotions connected with it. It is the aspect of *Pitta* that digests and metabolizes experiences and determines our reactions to them.

When in balance, *Sadhaka Pitta* promotes harmonious emotions, self-confidence, healthy desires, energy, motivation, passion and a feeling of fulfilment. When out of balance, it gives rise to negative emotions, including self-criticism, low self-esteem, mood swings, getting easily upset or angry, being overly analytical or judgmental, feeling aggressive, overambitious, jealous, snappy or sharp. *Pitta* types are likely to be aggravated at times of pressure, such as before exams, interviews and competitions, because they are highly competitive and fear failure. They have a tendency to suppress their emotions until their anger explodes. Crying and expressing themselves is important for *Pitta* types for the release of tension. They may get headaches,

Crying is important for Pitta *types, helping them to release their emotions.*

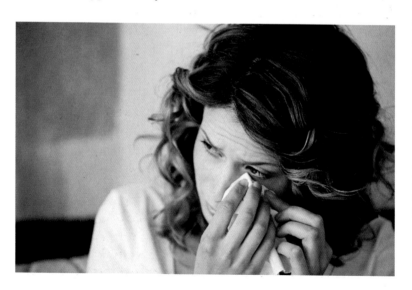

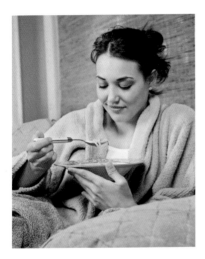

An excess of Tarpaka Kapha *might cause us to feel heavy and lethargic and to comfort-eat.*

sense of failure, which may lead to depression.

Pitta-type depression is not to be taken lightly. It can be deep and long-lasting. If left untreated, it can lead to serious depression, such as bipolar disease, suicidal tendencies or self-destructive behaviour such as abuse of drugs and alcohol, which only exacerbate the problem. It may lead to an imbalance in *Tarpaka Kapha* (see below), which is responsible for coordinating the heart and mind, causing further problems in the mind (*Prana Vata*), in which case all three *doshas* are disturbed.

Tarpaka Kapha

This is located in the brain, heart and cerebrospinal fluid. It provides nutrition, strength, protection and lubrication to the nerves. *Tarpaka* means 'contentment'. It has an inward movement, allowing us to feel the inner joy of being ourselves. In balance, *Tarpaka Kapha* gives us the light in the eyes, lustre of the skin, courage, fortitude,

burning sensations in the head and eyes and palpitations. Insomnia is a symptom of disturbed *Sadhaka Pitta*, but is different from *Vata* insomnia. *Pitta* people lie awake between 10 p.m. and 2 a.m., overburdened by responsibilities, with self-critical thoughts. They can be easily hurt and suffer from feelings of hopelessness and a

mental and emotional stability, resilience to stress, mental lucidity and *joie de vivre*. *Kapha* people are generally more placid and resilient, slower to react emotionally. Under stress they tend to become lethargic, withdrawn and lacking in motivation. They can become possessive, overly attached to people or things. They might eat more, and comfort-eating is likely. They put on weight easily and are reluctant to take exercise. They can sit for hours seemingly doing very little, perhaps watching television. Deficiency of *Tarpaka Kapha* can cause discontent, malaise, nervousness and insomnia, and symptoms of excess *Prana Vata*. Meditation promotes its secretion.

Balancing the *doshas*

The mind is a wonderful tool that we can use to obtain information from the world around us, with the help of the five senses. We have the ability to use our mind productively, but can also be at the mercy of its turbulent ways and may accumulate mental *Ama* (toxins) from undigested experiences and holding onto unresolved thoughts and negative emotions.

Balancing the *doshas* in a general way will help to remedy imbalances of specific aspects of them that relate to the mind and heart (see Chapter 12). Below are some guidelines for you.

Prana Vata

- Walk outdoors when the sun is rising, and breathe deeply. This helps open the channels, stimulates digestion and elimination, clearing any *Ama* from the previous day.
- Don't resist natural urges, as this can imbalance *Vata* and contribute to anxiety and emotional imbalance.
- Give yourself a daily *Abhyanga* (warm oil massage). The sense of touch is associated with emotions and helps balance *Vata* and calm anxiety and stress. Follow your massage with a warm

bath to flush out the toxins that have been pushed out from the cells during the massage.

• Use yoga *Asanas* or postures to enhance digestion, cleanse toxins from the channels and cells of the body that contribute to mental *Ama* and improve overall health.

• Inhale aromatic oils, including jatamansi, vetiver, frankincense, jasmine, rose and sandalwood.

• Perform *Pranayama* (breathing exercises).

Useful herbs: Tagarah, ashwagandha, rose, vacha, jatamansi, shankapushpi, shatavari, bringaraj, saffron, nutmeg, liquorice, black cumin, bala, kapikachu

Sadhaka Pitta

• Spend some time outside in a beautiful place in nature, especially by water.

Inhaling aromatic oils is a wonderful way to balance Prana Vata.

• Drink rose or chamomile tea when you need a calming drink.

• Avoid overexertion, both mental and physical.

• Massage daily with a cooling, relaxing oil, such as coconut or sesame oil, that contains essential oils of rose, chamomile, sandalwood, coriander or lemongrass.

• Listen to soothing, relaxing music, let go and relax.

• Go to bed before 10 p.m. Getting enough rest is essential for emotional health, and falling

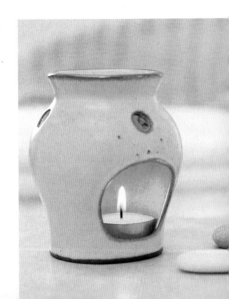

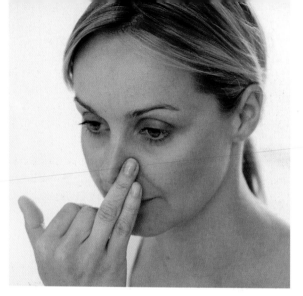

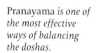
Pranayama *is one of the most effective ways of balancing the doshas.*

asleep during the *Kapha* time of night generates a deep, restful sleep that refreshes both mind and body.

Useful herbs: Rose, chamomile, amalaki, shatavari, bringaraj, aloe vera, manjishta, sariva, bacopa, gotu kola, jatamansi, shankapushpi, sandalwood, saffron, liquorice

Tarpaka Kapha

- Wake up with the rising sun. Waking after 6 a.m. causes the *srotas* (channels) to be clogged with *Ama*, leading to lethargy, dullness of mind, low moods and slow communication between heart and mind.
- Avoid sleeping in the daytime.
- Take plenty of vigorous exercise, do different things and try to be open-minded.
- Perform *Nasya*, or nasal administration of oils, including eucalyptus, nilyadi or vacha oil.

Useful herbs: Tulsi, rose, vacha, pippali, gotu kola, bacopa, frankincense, shankapushpi, saffron

Our mental and emotional constitution (*Manas Prakruti*)

The balance of the three *gunas* (*Sattva*, *Rajas* and *Tamas*) in our mental constitution has a profound effect on our state of mind and emotion (see Chapter 3).

There are three broad categories of mental *Prakrutis* (personalities). A person is called *Sattvic*, *Rajasic* or *Tamasic* according to the predominance of the *gunas* which in turn affect the three *doshas*. Although an interaction of all three is necessary, when *Sattva* (the quality of love, harmony and virtue) predominates it makes for the correct balance of all three *gunas*. When *Sattva*, *Rajas* and *Tamas* act together in unity, this balance is known as 'pure *Sattva*'.

The *Sattvic* mind

We can alter our *Manas Prakruti* through our thoughts, actions, diet, herbs and lifestyle. Ayurveda is primarily *Sattvic*, advocating a way of life with love, faith, peace, non-violence and other *Sattvic* virtues. By eating a healthy diet, and living a harmonious lifestyle with love, wisdom and other *Sattvic* attributes, we can experience a greater sense of peace, joy and fulfilment. Ayurveda recommends a code of physical conduct (*Svasthavitta*) and virtuous qualities (*Sdavritta*). This involves:

• A daily health regime (*Dinacharya*, see page 146) beginning with oil massage (*Abhyanga*) to remove toxins and stimulate the flow of natural intelligence in the body
• A seasonal health regime

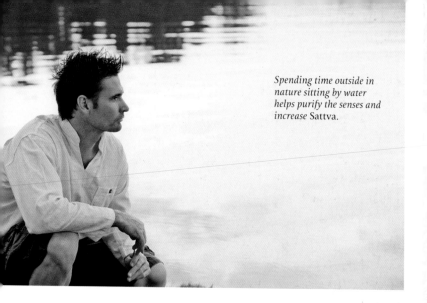

Spending time outside in nature sitting by water helps purify the senses and increase Sattva.

(*Rtucharya*, see page 204)

- Meditation to dissolve deep-rooted stress and promote harmony, creativity and clarity
- A healthy *Sattvic* diet in tune with your body type (see page 88)
- Regular exercise
- *Pranayama*
- Pure foods and water
- Avoiding toxins such as pesticides, alcohol and tobacco
- Purification or *Panchakarma* (see Chapter 17)
- Therapies such as Shirodhara and Marma massage (stimulation of the 107 Marma points to increase *Prana* and balance the *doshas*)
- Adequate sleep
- Spending time outside in nature, walking in the sunshine, sitting by water, to purify the senses
- A balance of activity and rest and relaxation, and time to reflect
- Being in loving, nurturing relationships
- Being kind and tolerant, and avoiding anger and criticism
- See also *Rasayana*, or rejuvenation therapy, in Chapter 18.

The role of meditation

According to the famous Indian doctor and Ayurvedic physician Deepak Chopra, 'The guiding principle of Ayurveda is that the mind exerts the deepest influence on the body, and freedom from sickness depends upon contacting our own awareness, bringing it into balance and extending that balance to the body.'

To help balance the mind and emotions, and eradicate the suffering that we experience in our state of disconnection from our inner source of light, we need to quieten the endless chatter in the mind and go within. Meditation can help to channel our awareness toward the inner self, and has the capacity to totally transform our state of mind, enabling union with the spirit. Through meditation we can observe the movements of the mind, thoughts, feelings and sensations as they come and go, by entering the awareness of the conscious witness. Since we can be observers of the mind, it means that we are not the mind – it is an instrument for our use.

The benefits of meditation

Daily meditation practice can also help clear mental and emotional *Ama* and prevent the build-up of more. When we feel anxious, fearful, upset or angry, a chain of physiological events is sparked off; hormones and biochemicals flood our bodies from the hypothalamus, pituitary and adrenal glands and have far-reaching effects throughout the body. In acute stress, our heart

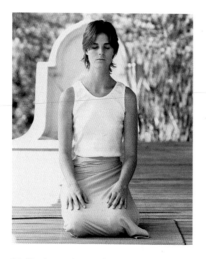

Meditation and repeating a mantra helps quieten the mind and harmonize our inner bodies.

depleting our *Ojas*, our vital energy and immunity. Research on meditation shows that it can increase *Ojas*, enhance our resilience to stress, reduce cortisol levels, lower blood pressure and negative emotions such as fear, aggression and anger. Even diseases caused by deep-seated *Ama*, such as heart disease, hypertension and stroke, are found to significantly improve with meditation.

There are many different forms of meditation, but common to all is the use of concentration techniques to help us witness our thoughts. Mantras – sounds, syllables, words or phrases (usually drawn from scripture and endowed with special power) – can be chanted to establish a force field. They can also be repeated softly or mentally, and their subtle tones will have the effect of quietening the mind, harmonizing the inner bodies and stimulating our latent spiritual qualities.

rate increases, blood flow to our muscles is increased, our pupils dilate and more oxygen flows through our lungs. In chronic stress, our bodies are in a state of hyper-arousal for long periods of time, and hormones that are meant to protect us are oversecreted, and eventually depleted. This has the effect of

Pranayama

Breathing exercises are known as *Pranayama*. *Prana* is the life force, and *Pranayama* increases *Agni*, opens and cleanses the mental channels (*Manovahasrotas*) that carry oxygen to the brain, and increases *Ojas*. It enhances mental clarity and balances the emotions.

It is best to practise *Pranayama* early in the morning in the fresh air. Below are some of the more popular exercises, which are generally done seated in a comfortable posture.

Bellow breath (*Bhastrika*)

This primarily consists of deep breathing, both in and out of the nose, with the emphasis on squeezing as much air out of the lungs as possible on the out-breath. Raise the shoulders when inhaling, to create more lung space. When you have repeated several breaths, this is known as a round. You can start with two rounds of five breaths, and gradually increase to rounds of 20 breaths. You generally finish a round by inhaling deeply, and then breathe normally again for two minutes before starting another round. If you feel dizzy, pause and then continue after a few normal breaths.

Bhastrika increases oxygenation, metabolism, blood circulation and heart function. It clears the nose and the mind and helps to release negative feelings such as anger, grief and depression. It is good for obesity, diabetes, high cholesterol, low thyroid function and muscle

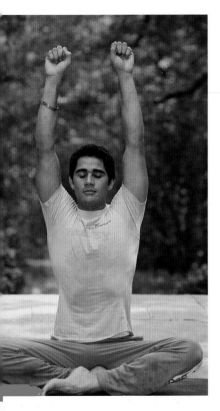

Pranayama is generally practised in the fresh air, early in the morning, seated in a comfortable posture.

pain. Avoid it with high blood pressure, after a recent heart attack, and when pregnant or menstruating.

Skull-shining breath (*Kapalabhati*)

Sit at the edge of your chair, take a deep breath in and then release the breath. Now inhale and exhale forcefully, breathing in and out rapidly, with the emphasis on the exhalation – a bit like blowing your nose.

The inhalation and abdominal movement will happen spontaneously. Finish by deep inhalation and exhalation. A beginner can do two rounds by doing 20 exhalations in each round. Take small breaks between each round. You can increase the number of exhalations and rounds as you feel ready, and can do up to 100 a minute.

Kapalabhati purifies the respiratory system and massages all the inner organs, bringing fresh blood to nourish them and aid

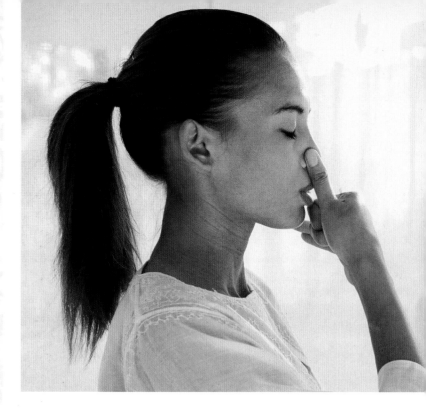

their function; 200–300 a day is good for the prostate, ovaries, formation of new blood cells, liver function, immunity and brain function. It boosts the supply of oxygen and purifies the blood, helps to tone up the abdominal muscles and reduce abdominal fat; it also clears anger and heat from

Alternate nostril breathing improves mental clarity and clears old mental and emotional patterns.

stagnant *Pitta* in the liver. Practise it before meditation as it improves concentration and helps to quieten the mind. Avoid during menstruation and pregnancy.

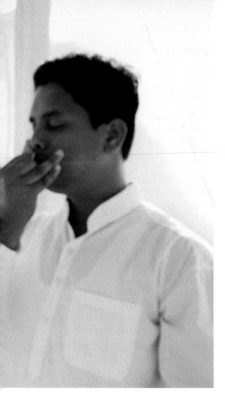

through your right nostril, replace your thumb over the right nostril and breathe out through your left nostril.

Repeating this 30 times in a round has the effect of balancing the right and left hemispheres of the brain, improving mental clarity, concentration and perception, and clearing old mental and emotional patterns. It also aids meditation.

Bee breath (*Brahmari*)

Sitting down, lift both arms and place each thumb over your ears, with your index fingers over the Third Eye in the centre of your forehead and the other fingers over your eyes. Breathe in deeply and, as you exhale, hum like a bee. This vibrates the throat, thyroid and heart, and helps keep them healthy.

Repeat this seven times initially, and work up to 17 repetitions. *Brahmari* is good for the pituitary and pineal glands and the endocrine system generally. It quietens the mind and benefits the eyes.

Alternate nostril breathing (*Anuloma Viloma*)

Place your right thumb over your right nostril and breathe in through the left nostril. Then close your left nostril with the ring finger of your right hand and breathe out through the right nostril. Then breathe in

281

Herbs for mental and emotional health

Herbs that have a nourishing and supportive effect on the mind, are known as *Medhya Rasayanas*. *Medhya* refers to the mind and intellect, while *Rasayana* is a tonic or rejuvenation therapy. These herbs enhance our memory and our concentration.

According to Ayurveda, mental ability is at its optimum when the three aspects of *Buddhi* – *dhi* (learning), *dhriti* (retention) and *smriti* (recall) – are working well individually and together. *Medhya Rasayanas* are good for enhancing each individual aspect of mental ability because they promote coordination among the cells, between mind and body and among the senses.

As nervine tonics, *Medhya Rasayanas* deeply nourish the neurological tissues, providing specific molecular nutrients for the brain, which can promote mental health and help alleviate mental, emotional and behavioural problems. In this way they have the ability to engender calmness and tranquillity. They have adaptogenic and rejuvenative effects, increasing resilience to stress and slowing the effects of ageing on the brain.

There is another category of herbs that have a supportive and rejuvenative effect on the heart and cardiovascular system, but also on the emotional heart, known as *Hridaya Rasayanas*. Just as *Medhya* herbs enhance mental and intellectual ability, so these amazing remedies enhance our ability to tolerate physical and emotional stress on the heart and flush out toxins that block the physical and mental channels.

THE BEST *MEDHYA RASAYANAS*

- **Ashwagandha** (*Withania somniferum*)
- **Brahmi** (*Bacopa monniera*)
- **Gotu kola** (*Centella asiatica*)
- **Shankapushpi** (*Evolvulus pluricaulis*)
- **Vacha** (*Acorus calamus*)
- **Shatavari** (*Asparagus racemosus*)
- **Krishna jiraka** (*Nigella sativa*)
- **Bala** (*Sida cordifolia*)
- **Kapikachu** (*Mucuna pruriens*)
- **Guduchi** (*Tinospora cordifolia*)
- **Bringaraj** (*Eclipta alba*)
- **Haritaki** (*Terminalia chebula*)
- **Liquorice** (*Glycyrrhiza glabra*)
- **Pippali** (*Piper longum*)
- **Rose** (*Rosa* sp.)

THE BEST *HRIDAYA RASAYANAS*

- **Arjuna** (*Terminalia arjuna*)
- **Amalaki** (*Emblica officinalis*)
- **Ashoka** (*Saraca indica*)
- **Bala** (*Sida cordifolia*)
- **Gotu kola** (*Centella asiatica*)
- **Guggulu** (*Commiphora mukul*)
- **Punarnava** (*Boerhavia diffusa*)
- **Tagarah** (*Valeriana wallichi*)
- **Tulsi** (*Ocimum sanctum*)
- **Vasaka** (*Adhatoda vasica*)
- **Cinnamon** (*Cinnamomum zeylanicum/cassia*)
- **Coriander** (*Coriandrum sativum*)
- **Rose** (*Rosa* sp.)

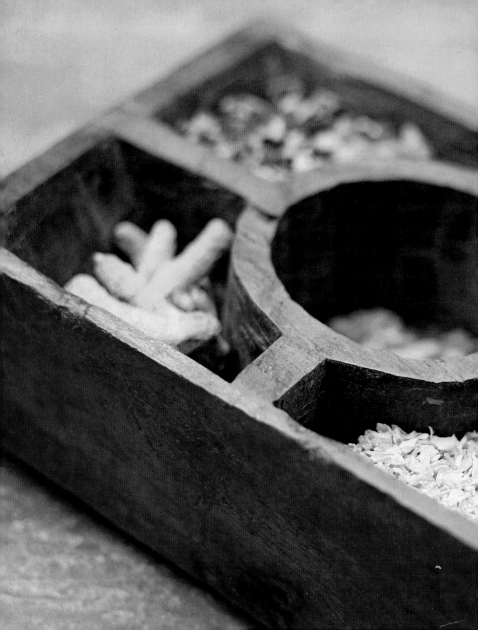

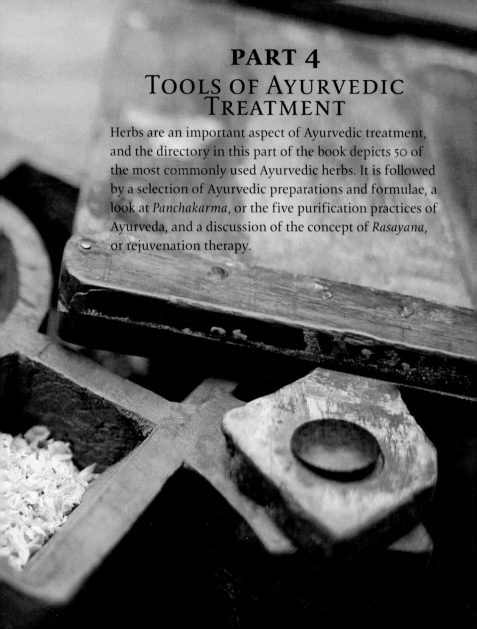

PART 4
TOOLS OF AYURVEDIC TREATMENT

Herbs are an important aspect of Ayurvedic treatment, and the directory in this part of the book depicts 50 of the most commonly used Ayurvedic herbs. It is followed by a selection of Ayurvedic preparations and formulae, a look at *Panchakarma*, or the five purification practices of Ayurveda, and a discussion of the concept of *Rasayana*, or rejuvenation therapy.

Chapter 15: **A directory of Ayurvedic herbs**

This directory describes in detail 50 herbs that are commonly used in Ayurvedic medicine. The herbs' botanical, Sanskrit and common names are given, followed by a summary of useful information: the parts of the plants that are used, and their quality, taste, potency and post-digestive effect; the predominant *dosha*, and the *dhatus* and *srotas* that are affected; a description of the herb's actions, a note on any cautions, and details of the relevant dosage.

A NOTE ON DOSAGES

Throughout this chapter the dosages are given in metric. Below are some simple conversions.

- 5 ml = 1 teaspoon, 15 ml = 1 tablespoon/½ fl oz, 25 ml = 1 fl oz, 100 ml = 3½ fl oz

- 3 gm = ½ teaspoon, 5 gm = 1 teaspoon/¼ oz, 15 gm = 1 tablespoon/½ oz, 25 gm = 1 oz, 50 gm = 2 oz

---

DOSHA ABBREVIATIONS

V: *Vata*

P: *Pitta*

K: *Kapha*

A minus sign after the abbreviation (e.g. P-) means the herb decreases the *dosha*; a plus sign (P+) means the herb increases it.

Ayurvedic herbs are described according to their qualities and tastes as well as their effects on the doshas, dhatus *and* srotas.

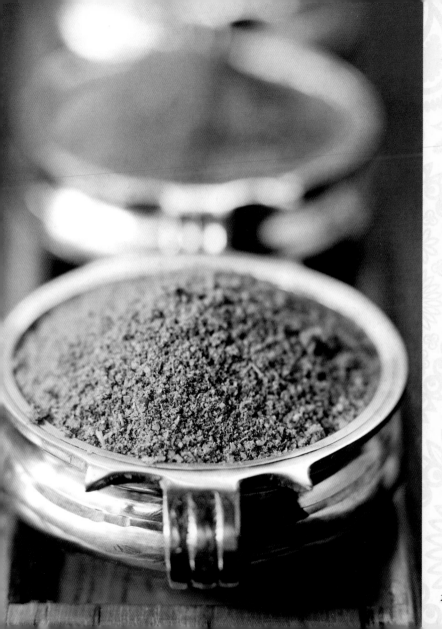

Acorus calamus

(Vacha, Sweet Flag)

Part used: rhizome
Quality: light, sharp, dry
Taste: bitter, pungent, astringent
Potency: heating
Post-digestive: pungent
Dosha: VK- P+
Dhatu: plasma, muscle, fat, nerve, reproductive
Srota: nervous, digestive, respiratory, circulatory, reproductive

ACTIONS

Nervine, antispasmodic, carminative, sedative, analgesic, expectorant, decongestant, emetic, laxative, diuretic, febrifuge, anti-inflammatory, antimicrobial, hypotensive, anticonvulsant, rejuvenative, stimulant.

A highly respected *Sattvic* tonic for the mind, vacha enhances mental clarity, concentration and speech. It clears the subtle channels of toxins and obstructions, promotes cerebral circulation and brain function. It is often combined with gotu kola to help meditation.

By stimulating *Agni*, vacha stimulates the appetite, digestion and absorption, and helps clear *Ama*. It is useful in obesity and to relieve colic, flatulence and peptic ulcers. Its antimicrobial and decongestant properties are helpful in infections in the gut, bronchitis, sinusitis, coughs, asthma and laryngitis. The oil is useful externally for painful arthritic joints. Taken nasally, it revitalizes *Prana*.

Cautions: It induces vomiting if taken in large doses.
Dosage: 1–5 gm powder, 1–5 ml tincture daily.

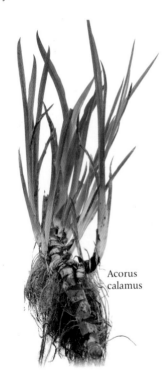

Acorus calamus

Adhatoda vasica

(Vasaka, Malabar Nut, Adusa)

Part used: root, leaves, flowers
Quality: light, dry
Taste: bitter, astringent
Potency: cold
Post-digestive: pungent
Dosha: KP- V+
Dhatu: plasma, blood, fat
Srota: respiratory, circulatory, digestive

ACTIONS

Bronchodilator, expectorant, astringent, antimicrobial, analgesic, anti-inflammatory, anti-allergenic, vasodilator, cardio-tonic, haemostatic, antispasmodic, alterative, styptic, uterine tonic, parturient, febrifuge.

Cooling and astringent, vasaka clears inflammation and heat from high *Pitta*, particularly in *Rakta dhatu*. It reduces nausea, diarrhoea and dysentery, heals ulcers and stops bleeding. In the lungs it clears congestion and relieves asthma, throat infections, coughs, fevers and allergies.

A tonic to the heart, vasaka lowers blood pressure and cleanses the blood. It clears *Kapha* toxins in *Rasa dhatu* and is helpful in inflammatory skin problems. It relieves urinary disorders and helps contract muscles, making it useful for uterine prolapse.

Cautions: Avoid during pregnancy (although it is useful a few weeks before childbirth as a parturient). Excess may cause hypotension. Best used under the guidance of a practitioner.
Dosage: 0.5–1.5 gm leaf powder/decoction 2–3 times daily

Aloe vera

(Kumari, Indian Aloe)

Part used: gel, leaves
Quality: oily, sticky
Taste: bitter, sweet, pungent, astringent
Potency: cooling
Post-digestive: sweet
Dosha: VPK= (P-)
Dhatu: all
Srota: digestive, excretory, circulatory, female reproductive

ACTIONS

Alterative, anti-inflammatory, anthelmintic, digestive, probiotic, laxative, bitter tonic, cholagogue, rejuvenative, immune-enhancing, antiviral, antitumour, emmenagogue, diuretic, demulcent, vulnerary.

The clear mucilaginous gel from inside the leaves has a cooling and soothing action in the body. When mixed with water, it makes the juice that is taken for problems associated with heat and inflammation, and is an excellent rejuvenative. It is particularly good for excess *Pitta* in the blood and for hot, fiery people, who are prone to inflammatory problems and feeling angry, irritable and self-critical.

A good bitter tonic for the liver and digestive tract, aloe juice enhances the secretion of digestive enzymes, balances stomach acid, aids digestion and regulates sugar and fat metabolism. It clears toxins, soothes and protects the gut lining, reduces pain and inflammation and has a mildly antibiotic effect. It supports the gut flora and helps combat harmful microorganisms in the stomach and bowel infections and dysbiosis. It can be used for colitis, peptic ulcers, diarrhoea, constipation, irritable bowel syndrome (IBS) and inflammatory bowel problems, including ulcerative colitis.

As a reproductive tonic, aloe juice regulates periods and relieves *Pitta* problems of heavy bleeding, clots, PMS and heat physically, as in hot flushes, and emotionally during the menopause.

Externally it may be applied to cuts, abrasions, allergic and inflammatory skin conditions. It heals burns, including sunburn and after radiation therapy. It is used in lotions to rejuvenate the skin and reduce wrinkles, and for haemorrhoids to soothe pain and speed healing. It also soothes inflammatory eye problems.

Cautions: The bitter, yellow juice from the rind of the leaves is a powerful laxative. Avoid in pregnancy, uterine bleeding and appendicitis. Occasionally it causes contact dermatitis. It may interact with cardiac glycosides.

Dosage: 30–60 ml juice daily

Aloe vera

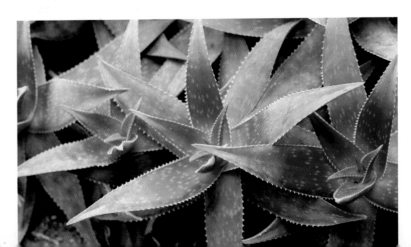

Andrographis paniculata

(Kalamegha, Kirata)

Part used: aerial parts
Quality: light, dry, penetrating
Taste: bitter, pungent
Potency: cooling
Post-digestive: pungent
Dosha: PK- V+
Dhatu: plasma, blood, fat
Srota: digestive, respiratory, circulatory, urinary

ACTIONS

Immunostimulant, anti-inflammatory, bitter tonic, cholagogue, hepatoprotective, febrifuge, anodyne, antimicrobial, antiviral, antifungal, antiparasitic and anthelmintic, antimalarial, antioxidant, probiotic, alterative.

Known as the 'king of bitters' for its very bitter taste, andrographis has wonderfully cooling and cleansing effects, clearing excess heat and *Pitta* from the blood. It is valued in Ayurveda for enhancing immunity, preventing and combating fevers, toxicity and acute infections. It can be taken for chest infections, pneumonia, tonsillitis, laryngitis, ear infections, colds, flu, sinusitis, Lyme's disease, leptospirosis, as well as post-viral problems, herpes, HIV,

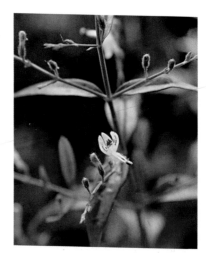

Andrographis paniculata

hepatitis A (and possibly B and C) and malaria. It may protect against cancer.

Andrographis is an excellent herb for the digestion. It enhances digestion and absorption, reduces inflammation, and relieves indigestion, flatulence, gastritis, colitis and peptic ulcers. It is especially good at cooling excess *Pachaka Pitta*, which can cause heat, heartburn, indigestion, acidity, burning and diarrhoea. It also helps re-establish normal gut flora and combats acute gastrointestinal infections, bacterial and amoebic dysentery, worms, parasites and candida. It stimulates bile flow from the liver, helps to digest fats, reduces high

Ranjaka Pitta and protects the liver against damage from toxins, alcohol and infection.

It lowers harmful LDL cholesterol and protects against atherosclerosis, heart disease and clots. By reducing *Pitta*, andrographis helps clear inflammation and infection in the urinary system. It is also excellent for hot, inflammatory skin conditions such as eczema, urticaria, acne, boils and abscesses.

Externally it may be used as a lotion/cream for inflamed and infected skin problems, as a douche/wash for vaginitis, and as a mouthwash/gargle for mouth ulcers, sore throats and gum disease.

Cautions: It has a possible antifertility effect. Avoid during pregnancy and high *Vata*. Use with caution with immunosuppressive drugs and anticoagulants.

Dosage: 1–6 gm dried herb daily as a powder or infusion

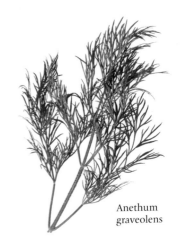

Anethum
graveolens

Anethum graveolens

(Sowa, Dill)

Part used: leaves, seeds
Quality: light, dry, penetrating
Taste: pungent, bitter
Potency: hot

Post-digestive: pungent
Dosha: VK- P+
Dhatu: plasma, muscle, nerve, reproductive
Srota: digestive, respiratory, female reproductive

ACTIONS

Carminative, expectorant, diuretic, antispasmodic, galactagogue, vermifuge, analgesic, relaxant, digestive, anti-inflammatory, antioxidant, antimicrobial, brain tonic, probiotic.

A well-known digestive, this highly aromatic herb stimulates the appetite, digestion and absorption, releases spasm and relieves colic, wind, indigestion, nausea, constipation and diarrhoea. In India it is used for worms. It helps re-establish normal gut flora, and is good for dysbiosis.

As a brain tonic, dill alleviates tiredness, but is also a good relaxant for *Vata*-type muscle tension and pain, insomnia and stress-related disorders, including painful periods and asthma. It is given to women before childbirth to ease contractions, and increases milk in breastfeeding women. With its diuretic effects, it soothes urinary-tract infections.

Dosage: 1–3 gm seed powder up to three times daily

Asparagus racemosus

(Shatavari, Wild Asparagus)

Part used: root
Quality: heavy, unctuous
Taste: sweet, bitter
Potency: cooling
Post-digestive: sweet
Dosha: VP- K+ (in excess)
Dhatu: all
Srota: digestive, female reproductive, respiratory

ACTIONS

Nutritive tonic, rejuvenative, galactagogue, adaptogenic, antispasmodic, nervine, anti-inflammatory, demulcent, refrigerant, diuretic, aphrodisiac, expectorant, antibacterial, alterative, antitumour, antacid, antidiarrhoetic.

An excellent nourishing tonic and the most important *Sattvic* rejuvenative for women, shatavari translates as 'she who possesses a hundred husbands'. It is cooling and moistening, restoring balance when the body and mind are overheated and depleted, soothing dry and inflamed mucous membranes in the respiratory tract, kidneys, stomach and sexual organs. It balances female hormones, increases fertility, relieves PMS, menstrual and menopausal problems and low libido, and increases milk supply during lactation.

Shatavari cools and soothes inflammatory problems in the digestive tract including acid indigestion, gastritis, peptic ulcers, inflammatory bowel

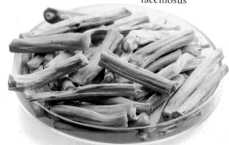

Asparagus racemosus

problems such as Crohn's disease and ulcerative colitis and, with its thirst-relieving and fluid-protecting powers, is good for chronic diarrhoea and dysentery. Soothing and cooling for cystitis, it dissolves stones and gravel and reduces fluid retention.

With its adaptogenic properties, shatavari enhances immunity, growth and development in babies and children. It stimulates white blood cells, helping to fight infection, and is a good antifungal for candida and thrush, antibacterial against a range of bacteria including salmonella, E-coli and pseudomonas and antiviral against herpes. It protects blood-producing cells in the bone marrow, aiding recovery after exposure to toxic chemicals. It is a good remedy for convalescence and is anti-inflammatory for gout and arthritis.

Shatavari has an affinity for the mind and is used to promote memory and mental clarity, and for ADHD in children, often combined with brain tonics such as gotu kola. It is calming, reduces anxiety and increases resilience to stress.

Externally, as an ingredient of Mahanaryan oil, it is used to reduce the development of scar tissue after surgery. It soothes the skin and eases *Vata* problems, including stiff and painful joints, stiff neck and muscle spasm.

Cautions: Avoid with high *Kapha*, low *Agni*, *Ama* and catarrh.

Dosage: 3–5 gm powder twice daily.

Azadirachta indica

(Nimba, Neem)

Part used: leaves, seeds, oil, bark
Quality: light, unctuous
Taste: bitter, astringent
Potency: cold
Post-digestive: pungent
Dosha: KP- V+ (in excess)
Dhatu: plasma, blood, fat, reproductive
Srota: circulatory, digestive, urinary, respiratory, reproductive

ACTIONS

Febrifuge, antiseptic, vulnerary, anthelmintic, insecticidal, alterative, anti-inflammatory, expectorant, bitter tonic, hepatoprotective, hypoglycaemic, antimalarial, antibacterial, antifungal, antiviral, astringent, antifertility, emmenagogue

Neem is one of the best antiseptic and detoxifying herbs of Ayurveda, excellent for combating infections and symptoms characterized by heat and inflammation.

Its bitter taste stimulates the appetite and digestion and increases bile flow from the liver. It enhances liver function and protects it from injury caused by toxins, drugs, chemotherapy and viruses. It is excellent for acidity, heartburn, indigestion, peptic ulcers, nausea and vomiting, bowel infections, dysbiosis and worms. It regulates the metabolism, aiding weight loss, and lowers blood sugar. Neem's cooling effect reduces 'heat' in the mind, relieving anxiety and stress, irritability, anger and depression. It reduces cholesterol and blood pressure and helps regulate the heart. It is used for inflammatory arthritis and for clearing skin problems, including eczema, acne, psoriasis, boils and abscesses.

Neem also helps clear infection and phlegm in coughs and chest infections, is used to reduce fevers and is excellent for the prevention and treatment of malaria. A decoction of the seeds is used in India for delayed and painful childbirth as it stimulates uterine contractions, and as a tonic after birth.

Externally the oil is excellent for skin problems and is widely used in non-toxic insecticides and in liniments for inflammatory joint and muscle pain.

Cautions: Avoid in pregnancy. It may reduce fertility and cause nausea and hypersensitivity reactions. Use with care in diabetic patients on insulin.

Dosage: 10–20 ml tincture of leaves daily, 2–4 gm powdered bark daily, 5–10 drops oil in a base oil for external use

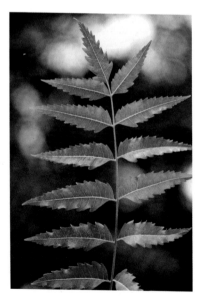

Bacopa monniera
(Brahmi, Bacopa)

Part used: aerial parts
Quality: light, flowing
Taste: bitter, sweet, astringent
Potency: cooling
Post-digestive: sweet
Dosha: VPK= V+ (in excess)
Dhatu: all, especially plasma, blood, nerve
Srota: digestive, nervous, circulatory, excretory

Azadirachta indica

ACTIONS

Adaptogen, antidepressant, nervine tonic, diuretic, sedative, cardio-tonic, rejuvenative, antispasmodic, carminative, bronchodilator, anticonvulsant, immunostimulant, anti-inflammatory, antiseptic, antifungal, antioxidant.

Brahmi derives its name from *Brahma*, meaning 'pure consciousness' because of its ability to calm mental turbulence and aid meditation. It is often confused with gotu kola (see page 299), which is also called Brahmi in northern India. Bacopa is considered a *Rasayana* (rejuvenative) for the brain and nerve tissue and is particularly good for relieving *Vata* disorders and disturbance of *Sadhaka Pitta*. It is wonderful for improving brain function and learning capacity, increasing concentration and memory, and is used as a remedy for epilepsy, anxiety, insomnia, learning problems including ADD, ADHD and Asperger's syndrome, Alzheimer's, Parkinson's disease, dementia, agitation and mental illness. It increases resilience to stress, combats nervous exhaustion and relieves depression. It is also used for low thyroid function.

Bacopa can also be used in prescription for coughs and colds, bronchitis and asthma, and acts as a cooling diuretic for relieving cystitis and an irritable bladder. It makes a good relaxing remedy for stress-related diarrhoea, constipation and irritable bowel syndrome, since it can suppress appetite, it is best combined with warming digestive herbs such as ginger or cardamom. It is cleansing as it helps chelate (remove from the bloodstream by binding to) heavy metals from the body. It aids stress-related skin problems such as eczema, and its anti-inflammatory properties relieve joint pain.

Externally the oil or fresh leaf juice/paste can be applied to joints to relieve pain, and to the head to clear the mind and relieve headaches.

Cautions: Large doses may increase blood pressure.

Dosage: two cups infusion daily, 2.5–5 ml drops tincture twice a day, 2 gm powder twice a day

Bacopa monniera

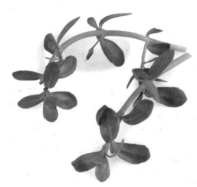

Bauhinia variegata

(Kanchanara, Mountain Ebony)

Part used: bark
Quality: dry, light
Taste: bitter, astringent
Potency: cooling
Post-digestive: pungent
Dosha: KP- V+
Dhatu: blood, muscle, fat, bone, reproductive
Srota: reproductive, excretory

ACTIONS

Alterative, lymphatic, astringent, anti-inflammatory, haemostatic, bone tonic, vulnerary, uterine tonic, antispasmodic, expectorant.

With its affinity for *Meda dhatu*, kanchanara is excellent for swollen glands, swellings and growths associated with excess *Kapha*. It has a detoxifying action and helps clear inflammatory skin problems. It is specific for gynaecological problems associated with excess *Kapha*, including fibroids, cysts, polycystic ovaries and endometriosis. It reduces heavy bleeding.

It makes a good astringent for diarrhoea, haemorrhoids and prolapse. By reducing *Avalambaka Kapha*, it reduces catarrh and clears coughs. With its affinity for *Asthi dhatu* it can be used for osteoporosis. A decoction can be used as a gargle for sore throats.

Cautions: Avoid during pregnancy and with constipation.
Dosage: 1–10 gm powder daily, 3–15 ml tincture daily

Bauhinia variegata

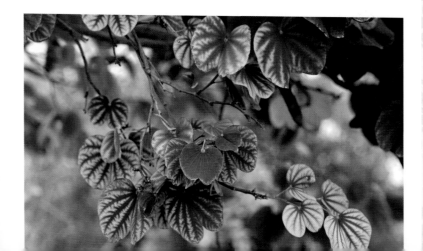

Boerhavia diffusa

(Punarnava, Indian Hogweed)

Part used: whole plant
Quality: dry, light
Taste: bitter, sweet
Potency: cooling
Post-digestive: pungent
Dosha: VKP- V+ (in excess)
Dhatu: plasma, blood, fat, nerve, reproductive
Srota: urinary, digestive, circulatory

ACTIONS

Alterative, blood tonic, diuretic, rejuvenative, kidney tonic, digestive, carminative, hypoglycaemic, anthelmintic, astringent, antihaemorrhagic.

A famous rejuvenative, Punarnava increases *Ojas*, strengthens the kidneys and boosts energy and vitality. It is good for fluid retention associated with excess *Kapha*, bladder infections, kidney stones, oedema from poor cardiac function, and breathlessness. It stimulates the digestion and relieves colic, wind and diarrhoea. It curbs heavy menstrual bleeding. By reducing *Meda dhatu* it can be used for diabetes and obesity.

It is helpful for swollen watery joints, arthritis and gout, as it moves toxins and fluid from the joints and tissues and aids their elimination via the kidneys.

Cautions: Use with care in cases of dehydration, and with sedative, antidepressive and antiepileptic drugs. It may potentiate ACE inhibitors.
Dosage: 250–500 mg powder daily, 3–15 ml tincture daily

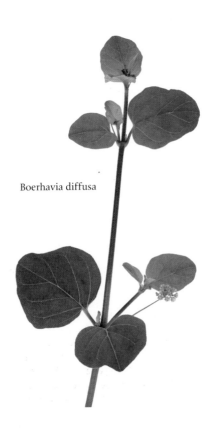

Boerhavia diffusa

Boswellia serrata

(Shallaki, Frankincense)

Part used: gum resin
Quality: dry, light, penetrating
Taste: bitter, pungent, sweet, astringent
Potency: heating and cooling
Post-digestive: pungent
Dosha: VKP=
Dhatu: all
Srota: circulatory, nervous, reproductive, musculoskeletal

ACTIONS

Anti-inflammatory, alterative, antispasmodic, analgesic, anti-arthritic, anti-tumour, aphrodisiac, decongestant, reduces cholesterol, vulnerary.

Frankincense clears toxins, speeds healing and reduces swelling and pain in rheumatoid and osteoarthritis, tendonitis, bursitis, repetitive strain injuries, gout, muscle pain and spasm, nerve pain and multiple sclerosis, as well as inflammatory gut problems, such as Crohn's disease and ulcerative colitis.

It reduces cholesterol, strengthens the blood vessels and improves blood flow to the joints and reproductive tissue, improving erectile and sexual function, and relieves uterine congestion, fibroids, cysts and painful periods with clots.

Frankincense also clears the airways and relieves catarrh, coughs, bronchitis and asthma. It deepens the breathing, opens the mind and also has a meditative effect.

Externally it may be used on wounds and bruises, piles and skin problems such as boils, psoriasis and urticaria.
Cautions: Avoid in pregnancy.
Dosage: 250 mg–1 gm purified powder daily

Centella/Hydrocotyle asiatica

(Mandukaparni, Brahmi, Gotu Kola)

Part used: aerial parts
Quality: light, dry
Taste: sweet, bitter, astringent
Potency: cooling
Post-digestive: sweet
Dosha: VPK=
Dhatu: plasma, blood, muscle, fat, bone, nerve
Srota: nervous, circulatory, digestive, muscular, reproductive

ACTIONS

Nerve tonic, anticonvulsant, analgesic, sedative, brain tonic, cardio-tonic, immunostimulant, febrifuge, alterative, diuretic, anthelmintic, vulnerary, rejuvenative, hair tonic.

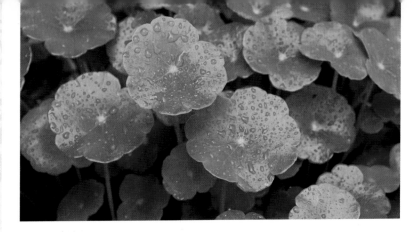

Centella asiatica

Gotu kola enhances memory and concentration and protects against the ageing process and Alzheimer's. It is excellent for high *Sadhaka Pitta* and children with learning difficulties, such as ADHD, autism and Asperger's. It relieves stress and anxiety, insomnia and depression and calms mental turbulence. It supports the adrenal glands and helps rebuild energy reserves.

Gotu kola strengthens immunity and helps fight off infections, including *Pseudomonas, Streptococcus* and *Herpes simplex*. Its detoxifying and anti-inflammatory properties are excellent for arthritis, gout and skin problems such as eczema, psoriasis, herpes, boils and acne. It relieves nervous indigestion, acidity and ulcers.

Gotu kola is an important herb for the circulation. After trauma such as surgery it stimulates microcirculation to the area and speeds healing. It promotes hair and nail growth, increases the tensile integrity of the skin, reduces cellulite and protects the skin against radiation. It prevents bleeding and is helpful in anaemia. It is used for oedema, venous insufficiency, varicose veins and anal fissures.

Externally the fresh juice or a poultice/decoction of dried leaves speeds the healing of wounds, burns, keloid scars, cervicitis, vaginitis, varicose veins and ulcers, and haemorrhoids. When prepared in coconut oil, it can be applied to the head to calm the mind, promote sleep, relieve headaches and prevent hair loss; it is applied to the skin in eczema and herpes.

Cautions: It can potentiate the action of anxiolytics (drugs used to treat anxiety).

Dosage: 50–100 ml (2–4 fl oz) infusion twice daily, 1–3 gm powder twice daily

Cinnamomum zeylanicum/cassia

(Twak, Cinnamon)

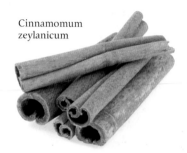

Cinnamomum zeylanicum

Part used: inner bark, oil
Quality: dry, light, penetrating
Taste: pungent, sweet, astringent
Potency: warming
Post-digestive: sweet
Dosha: VK- P+ (in excess)
Dhatu: plasma, blood, muscle, nerve, reproductive
Srota: respiratory, digestive, nervous, circulatory, urinary, reproductive

ACTIONS

Antimicrobial, antioxidant, aphrodisiac, tonic, immunostimulant, nervine, analgesic, mood-elevating, adaptogenic, circulatory stimulant, antispasmodic, astringent, digestive, diaphoretic, carminative, alterative, expectorant, diuretic, reduces cholesterol.

A wonderfully warming and delicious-tasting tonic for combating infections and improving digestion, cinnamon increases *Ojas* and is almost a universal panacea. It is *Sattvic* and excellent for *Vata* problems, improving resistance to stress, relieving fatigue and low spirits, tension and anxiety, as well as headaches and toothache. It improves memory, concentration and motivation.

Cinnamon enhances digestion and absorption, and relieves indigestion, anorexia, colic, nausea, bloating and wind from low *Agni*. Its astringent properties protect the gut lining against irritation and infection, inflammation and ulcers, and combat diarrhoea, dysentery, candida and dysbiosis. It enhances the effectiveness of insulin, helping prevent and improve diabetes.

It stimulates the circulation, relieves Raynaud's disease, increases blood flow to the joints (thereby helping to improve arthritis) and lowers cholesterol. It clears *Vata* and *Kapha* from the lungs. Taken hot, it helps throw off bacterial and viral infections, fevers, colds, catarrh, coughs and chest infections. It strengthens the kidneys and relieves cystitis and urinary-tract infections.

Rich in magnesium, cinnamon helps maintain bone density and hormone balance. It is good for PMS, irregular, painful and heavy periods, and as a reproductive tonic aids low libido, impotence, ovarian cysts, fibroids, endometriosis and infections, including thrush.

Externally it may be used in inhalations as a decongestant for colds, sore throats, coughs, sinusitis and catarrh; in oil massage for tense, aching muscles; and as a wash for cuts, wounds, bites, stings and infective skin problems.

Cautions: Avoid in pregnancy, and cases of high *Pitta*.

Dosage: 1–10 gm bark/powder daily, 3–15 ml tincture daily

Commiphora mukul
(Guggulu, Indian Myrrh)

Part used: gum resin
Quality: light, dry, penetrating
Taste: bitter, pungent
Potency: heating
Post-digestive: pungent
Dosha: VPK= P+ (in excess)
Dhatu: all
Srota: digestive, respiratory, circulatory, nervous

ACTIONS
Anti-inflammatory, alterative, nervine, antispasmodic, analgesic, expectorant, astringent, cardio-tonic, lowers cholesterol, antioxidant, diaphoretic, antimicrobial, immunostimulant, rejuvenative, vulnerary, thyroid stimulant, emmenagogue, metabolic regulator.

An honoured Ayurvedic remedy for scraping toxins out of the body and lowering harmful cholesterol, guggulu is a wonderful rejuvenative, particularly for *Vata* and *Kapha*. It inhibits the formation of clots and reduces atherosclerosis, helps prevent heart disease and angina, and reduces the risk of stroke and pulmonary embolism. It is excellent for boosting immunity. It increases white blood-cell count, helping to combat infections, and disinfects secretions, including sweat, mucus and urine. Its antimicrobial and antispasmodic properties are helpful in coughs, chest infections and whooping cough.

Guggulu is a good anti-inflammatory and cleansing remedy for gout and

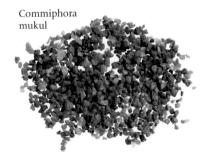

Commiphora mukul

arthritis, lumbago and sciatica. It is traditionally used for healing fractures and deep-seated wounds, as well as for regenerating nerve tissue. It reduces inflammation in acute and chronic skin disease, including nodulocystic acne, and enhances healing.

It is an excellent herb for the reproductive system. It has the ability to break down growths and tumours such as lipomas, and has an affinity for the lower abdomen, reducing fibroids, cysts, endometriosis and polycystic ovarian syndrome. It helps regulate the cycle and prevent clotting.

Guggulu is one of the best herbs for digestion and metabolism, especially fat metabolism, and helps to reduce overweight and obesity by regulating the thyroid gland. It can reduce blood sugar in diabetes.

Externally guggulu may be used as a gargle for tonsillitis and mouth ulcers, and as a lotion/cream for eczema and acne.

Cautions: It can reduce the effect of anti-hypertensives such as Propranolol and Diltiazem; use with caution with hypoglycaemic medication. Avoid in acute kidney infections, excessive uterine bleeding, thyrotoxicosis, pregnancy and breastfeeding.

Dosage: two tablets two or three times daily

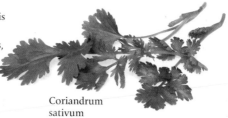

Coriandrum
sativum

Coriandrum sativum

(Dhanya, Coriander)

Part used: seeds, leaves
Quality: light, oily
Taste: sweet, bitter, pungent
Potency: cooling
Post-digestive: sweet
Dosha: VPK=
Dhatu: plasma, blood, muscle, nerve, reproductive
Srota: digestive, nervous, urinary, respiratory

ACTIONS

Carminative, digestive, antimicrobial, diuretic, decongestant, antispasmodic, antioxidant, alterative, nervine, rejuvenative, aphrodisiac, analgesic, diaphoretic.

Coriander seeds are antimicrobial, and the fresh leaves are rich in antioxidant vitamins and minerals and draw out toxins. This herb cools hot, inflammatory *Pitta* conditions, headaches, migraine, muscle pain and neuralgia. Coriander promotes mental clarity, improves mood and memory, and relieves lethargy and anxiety.

Coriander eases period pain, PMS and hot flushes. In hot tea the seeds combat eruptive infections, fevers, colds, flu, coughs and catarrh, allergies such as eczema and hay fever, and urinary disorders. Coriander enhances the digestion and absorption, and relieves griping, wind, heartburn and nervous indigestion.

Externally, leaf juice/tea soothes inflamed skin, and may be used as a gargle for sore throats and thrush, or as a lotion for conjunctivitis.

Dosage: 3–6 gm powder daily

Cuminum cyminum

(Jeera, Cumin)

Part used: seeds
Quality: dry, light
Taste: bitter, pungent
Potency: cooling
Post-digestive: pungent
Dosha: VPK= P+ (in excess)
Dhatu: plasma, blood, muscle, reproductive
Srota: digestive, respiratory, reproductive

ACTIONS

Carminative, digestive, decongestant, alterative, antispasmodic, diuretic, galactagogue.

Well known for its digestive properties, cumin enhances the appetite, digestion and absorption and clears toxins from the gut. It relieves wind, bloating and poor digestion from excess *Vata* and *Kapha*. It is particularly good for nausea and indigestion from upward-moving *Vata* as it redirects *Apana Vata* downward. It is also good for diarrhoea as it absorbs fluids from the large intestine.

Cuminum cyminum

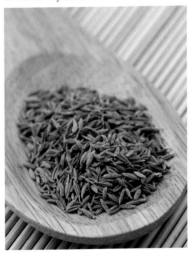

Cumin clears excess *Avalambaka Kapha* from the lungs, relieving catarrh, coughs, chest infections and asthma. It has an affinity with the female reproductive system, reducing pain and inflammation and enhancing the production of breast milk in nursing mothers, particularly when combined with shatavari.

Dosage: 0.5–6 gm powder daily, 3–15 ml tincture daily

Curcuma longa
(Haldi, Turmeric)

Part used: rhizomes
Quality: dry, light
Taste: pungent, bitter, astringent
Potency: hot
Post-digestive: pungent
Dosha: VPK= PV+ (in excess)
Dhatu: all
Srota: digestive, circulatory, respiratory, reproductive

ACTIONS

Antioxidant, anti-inflammatory, alterative, digestive, analgesic, stimulant, carminative, vulnerary, antibacterial, lowers cholesterol, prevents clotting.

A great aid to digestion (particularly of protein and fats), turmeric promotes absorption and metabolism and helps weight loss. It enhances liver function, aids detoxification and protects the liver against damage from toxins. As a probiotic, it regulates the intestinal flora and can be used after antibiotics and for candida, worms, indigestion, heartburn, wind, bloating, colic and diarrhoea. It soothes the gut lining, protecting it against the effects of stress, excess acid, drugs and other irritants, and reducing the risk of gastritis and ulcers. It lowers blood sugar in diabetics.

Turmeric is excellent for the immune system, warding off infections such as colds, sore throats, coughs and fevers. It is good for skin problems such as acne and psoriasis, and for kidney and bladder problems. As a powerful antioxidant, it protects against free-radical damage and cancer, especially of the colon and breast. It enhances the production of cancer-fighting cells, and helps to protect against environmental toxins and the toxic effects of cigarettes.

Turmeric lowers cholesterol levels and inhibits blood-clotting, helping to prevent heart and arterial disease. It is a powerful anti-inflammatory, excellent for arthritis. It is valued by those who practise yoga for its beneficial effect on the ligaments.

Externally the powder, mixed with water or aloe-vera gel, can be applied to insect bites, inflamed and infected skin

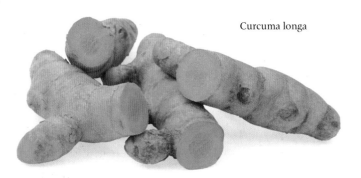

Curcuma longa

problems and wounds. It reduces itching, relieves pain and promotes healing in skin cancer, and slows ageing. You can also use it as a mouthwash for inflamed gums and toothache.

Cautions: Avoid large doses in pregnancy, with peptic ulcers and gall stones. Use with care with anticoagulants and non-steroidal anti-inflammatories.

Dosage: 1–10 gm powder daily, 5–15 ml tincture daily

Cymbopogon citratus

(Bhu Trna, Lemongrass)

Part used: leaves
Quality: dry, light, penetrating
Taste: bitter, pungent, sour
Potency: cooling

Post-digestive: pungent
Dosha: VPK= V+ (in excess)
Dhatu: plasma, blood, muscle, nerve
Srota: digestive, respiratory, urinary, female reproductive

ACTIONS

Digestive, febrifuge, analgesic, expectorant, anti-inflammatory, emmenagogue, antispasmodic, diuretic, galactagogue, decongestant, anthelmintic.

Lemongrass raises *Agni* and clears *Ama*, enhancing the digestion without aggravating *Pitta* because it is cooling. It regulates *Samana Vata* and *Apana Vata* and eases wind, bloating, abdominal pain and cramps, and worms.

Lemongrass relieves period pain from excess *Vata* or *Pitta* and enhances milk production. It makes a soothing diuretic for cystitis and fluid retention. It reduces *Avalambaka Kapha* in the lungs, clears phlegm in coughs and bronchitis, and eases spasms and congestion in asthma. In hot infusions it reduces fevers.

Externally the oil increases circulation and relieves the pain and inflammation of arthritic joints. It may be applied to skin problems and alopecia.

Dosage: 1–9 gm powder daily, 5–15 ml tincture daily.

Cyperus rotundus

(Musta, Mustaka, Nut Grass)

Part used: root
Quality: dry, light
Taste: bitter, pungent, astringent
Potency: cooling
Post-digestive: pungent
Dosha: PKV= V+ (in excess)
Dhatu: plasma, blood, muscle, nerve
Srota: digestive, circulatory, reproductive

ACTIONS

Carminative, emmenagogue, probiotic, alterative, astringent, anthelmintic, analgesic, febrifuge, digestive, galactagogue, hormone-balancing.

A great digestive for raising *Agni* and clearing *Ama* without aggravating *Pitta*, musta regulates *Samana Vata* and *Apana Vata*, relieving pain, spasm, wind, bloating, poor digestion and absorption and diarrhoea. It helps re-establish the gut flora, combats dysbiosis and soothes inflammation. With its affinity for *Ranjaka Pitta* in the liver, musta enhances bile secretion, metabolism and detoxification.

It is excellent for fevers as it clears heat and *Ama* from *Rasa dhatu* and *Rakta dhatu* and regulates *Agni*. It reduces painful periods, breast pain and PMS. It purifies and nourishes breast milk.

Dosage: 0.5–12 gm powder daily, 3–15 ml tincture daily

Cyperus rotundus

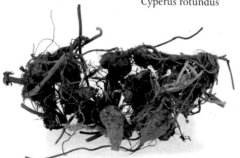

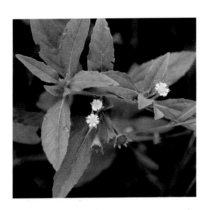

Eclipta alba

Eclipta alba

(Bringaraj, False Daisy)

Part used: leaves
Quality: light, dry
Taste: pungent, bitter, sweet
Potency: cooling
Post-digestive: pungent
Dosha: VPK= P *Rasayana*
Dhatu: plasma, blood, bone, nerve, reproductive
Srota: digestive, nervous, circulatory, respiratory, urinary, reproductive

ACTIONS

Liver tonic and protective, hypotensive, alterative, purgative, antioxidant, antimicrobial, rejuvenative, febrifuge, anti-inflammatory, haemostatic, anthelmintic.

A superb rejuvenative, bringaraj has antioxidant properties, increasing longevity and protecting against the ageing process. It improves memory and concentration, and helps to prevent age-related mental decline and Alzheimer's, as well as premature greying of the hair and balding. It is traditionally used for vertigo, declining eyesight and hearing.

Excellent for disturbances of *Sadhaka Pitta*, bringaraj reduces blood pressure and eases nervous palpitations. It calms nervous tension and anxiety and is helpful in irritability and anger, insomnia and mental agitation from high *Pitta* or *Vata*. It is also used for anaemia.

It has cooling and anti-inflammatory effects and benefits many *Pitta* symptoms characterized by heat. Its antimicrobial and decongestant properties help combat respiratory infections and catarrh.

Bringaraj improves digestion and absorption, and aids elimination of toxins by stimulating the bowels. It enhances the flow of bile from the liver and is excellent for liver problems, including cirrhosis and hepatitis. It protects the liver against damage from infection, drugs, chemicals and alcohol, and aids the liver in its cleansing work. It is beneficial for skin problems, including urticaria, eczema, psoriasis and vitiligo, reducing itching and inflammation, and is said to promote a lustrous complexion. It strengthens bone tissue and helps prevent tooth loss.

Externally the oil, which is prepared by boiling fresh leaves with coconut or sesame oil, promotes healthy hair, helps prevent baldness and greying, and soothes inflammatory skin conditions. The leaf juice is applied to minor cuts, abrasions and burns.

Dosage: 5–10 ml fresh juice three times daily, 3–5 gm powder twice daily

Eletteria cardamomum

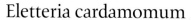

(Ela, Cardamom)

Part used: seed
Quality: light, dry
Taste: pungent, sweet
Potency: heating
Post-digestive: pungent
Dosha: VK- P+ (in excess)
Dhatu: plasma, blood, nerve
Srota: digestive, respiratory, circulatory, nervous

ACTIONS

Carminative, antispasmodic, decongestant, expectorant, diaphoretic, digestive, mild laxative, circulatory stimulant, nervine.

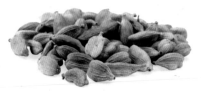

Eletteria
cardamomum

Cardamom lifts the spirits and induces a calm, meditative state. It eases tension and anxiety, lethargy and nervous exhaustion, and improves memory and concentration. Warming and invigorating, it also improves digestion and absorption, and relieves muscle pain and spasm. It eases stress-related digestive problems, indigestion, colic, wind, constipation, nausea, vomiting and travel sickness. It counteracts excess acidity and prevents drowsiness after eating.

This spice soothes sore throats and clears catarrh and is used for colds, coughs, asthma and chest infections. It enhances the circulation and increases energy. It strengthens a weak bladder, helping incontinence and bedwetting in children, as well as urinary-tract infections.

Externally the oil may be used in a massage oil for joint pain.

Cautions: Use with care with gastro-oesophageal reflux and gall stones.
Dosage: two tablets twice or three times daily, or 50–100 ml hot infusion

Emblica officinalis/ Phyllanthus emblica

(Amalaki, Indian Gooseberry)

Part used: fruit
Quality: light, dry
Taste: sweet, sour, pungent, bitter, astringent
Potency: cooling
Post-digestive: sweet
Dosha: VPK=
Dhatu: all
Srota: digestive, excretory, circulatory

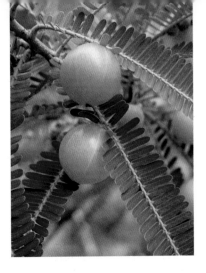

Emblica officinalis

ACTIONS

Antimicrobial, cooling, rejuvenative, antioxidant, hepatoprotective, lowers cholesterol, anti-inflammatory, laxative, hypoglycaemic, digestive, nutritive, diuretic.

A wonderful tonic, especially for *Pitta*, amalaki relieves heat, inflammation and burning throughout the body. Its cleansing and nourishing properties help purify the blood, rebuild tissues after injury or illness, improve eyesight and relieve allergies. It strengthens the teeth and bones and promotes the growth of hair and nails. It is good for anaemia as it stops bleeding and increases red blood-cell count.

Amalaki enhances digestion and absorption and is good for peptic ulcers, acidity, anorexia, nausea, vomiting,

gastritis, colitis and piles. It is an ingredient of the bowel-cleanser Triphala, for constipation and IBS. Its antioxidant properties protect the liver and it also regulates blood sugar. It is used with lemon juice in acute dysentery, and with fenugreek seeds in chronic diarrhoea.

Famous for relieving debility following illness, stress or in old age, amalaki is the main ingredient of Chayawanprash, which is a brain tonic, improving memory and concentration and calming anger and irritability. It reduces cholesterol and helps prevent clotting, protecting the cardiovascular system.

Amalaki enhances immunity. It has antimicrobial activity against viruses, bacteria and fungi, and helps combat candida, coughs, colds, flu, chest infections, asthma and urinary-tract infections. It may slow the growth of cancer cells.

Externally it is used in hair oils/soaps to prevent hair loss and as a skincare ingredient against oxidative damage.
Dosage: 5–30 gm powder daily, 5–15 ml tincture daily

Evolvulus alsinoides

(Shankapushpi)

Part used: leaves
Quality: unctuous, light
Taste: bitter, pungent, astringent
Potency: cooling
Post-digestive: sweet
Dosha: VPK=
Dhatu: plasma, nerve, reproductive
Srota: nervous, excretory, reproductive

ACTIONS

Nervine, sedative, brain tonic, laxative, vulnerary, haemostatic, digestive, antispasmodic.

Shankapushpi is one of the best brain tonics and calming herbs, excellent for nervous disorders, including pain, anxiety, insomnia, dizziness and convulsions. With its downward-moving action it rebalances *Apana Vata*, improves digestion and elimination. It is used for stress-related digestive problems such as colic and constipation. It helps to stop bleeding in the digestive, urinary and reproductive systems. As a reproductive tonic, it is used to promote fertility.

With its cleansing properties shankapushpi purifies the blood and helps clears the skin, especially in stress-related skin problems.
Cautions: It may potentiate sedative medication.
Dosage: 2–10 gm dried daily, 3–15 ml tincture daily

Evolvulus alsinoides

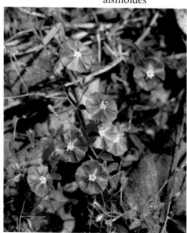

Ferula asafoetida

(Hing, Asafoetida)

Part used: seeds
Quality: sharp, hot and unctuous
Taste: bitter, pungent
Potency: heating
Post-digestive: pungent
Dosha: VK- P+
Dhatu: plasma, blood, muscle, bone, nerve
Srota: digestive, respiratory, nervous, excretory, circulatory, reproductive

ACTIONS

Carminative, digestive, anthelmintic, antispasmodic, diuretic, analgesic, emmenagogue, expectorant, cardiac stimulant.

Strengthening and calming, asafoetida is excellent for *Vata*. Taken before meals, it improves the appetite and digestion and relieves bloating, wind, constipation and colic. It balances the gut flora.

By regulating *Apana Vata* it eases nervous conditions, such as pain, cramps, tense muscles, sciatica, exhaustion and convulsions. It is excellent for coughs, asthma, fevers and whooping cough.

It stimulates blood flow to the uterus and regulates menstruation. It is good for painful periods, low libido, impotence and infertility, and for urinary problems, including cystitis. It reduces *Kapha* congestion and is cleansing after childbirth.

Externally it may be applied on the genitalia for impotence.
Cautions: Use with care with *Pitta*, inflammation of the liver, and pregnancy.
Dosage: 100 mg–1 gm powder or 1–3 ml tincture 3 times daily

Ferula asafoetida

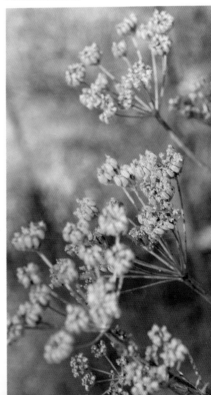

Foeniculum vulgare

(Madhurika, Fennel)

Part used: seeds
Quality: dry, light
Taste: bitter, pungent, sweet
Potency: cooling
Post-digestive: sweet
Dosha: VPK= P+ (in excess)
Dhatu: plasma, blood, muscle, nerve
Srota: digestive, respiratory, urinary, nervous, reproductive

ACTIONS

Carminative, digestive, antispasmodic, diuretic, galactagogue, expectorant, emmenagogue.

Fennel improves *Agni* without aggravating *Pitta*, and soothes inflammatory conditions, especially when combined with liquorice. It clears toxins, redirects the flow of *Apana Vata* downward, and relieves indigestion, wind, nausea, vomiting, bloating, cramps and piles. Chewing the seeds after eating settles the digestion and prevents wind and distension.

Its diuretic effects cool *Pitta*, relieve oedema and cystitis, and help clear inflamed skin and fevers.

Fennel also nourishes the brain and the eyes, and is excellent when tense muscles restrict the flow of *Vata*. It reduces *Kapha* congestion in the chest, relieving coughs and asthma. It brings on menstruation, relieves period pain and increases the flow of breast milk.

Dosage: 500 mg–9 gm powder daily, 3–15 ml tincture daily

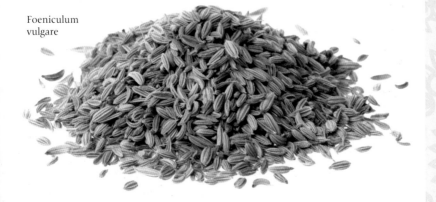

Foeniculum
vulgare

Glycyrrhiza glabra

(Yastimadhu, Liquorice)

Part used: peeled roots and runners
Quality: heavy, moist
Taste: sweet, bitter
Potency: sweet
Post-digestive: cooling
Dosha: VPK= K+ (in excess)
Dhatu: all
Srota: digestive, respiratory, nervous, excretory, reproductive

ACTIONS

Demulcent, expectorant, tonic, laxative, emetic, anti-inflammatory, febrifuge, diuretic, adaptogen, adrenal tonic, rejuvenative, sedative, hepatoprotective, antacid.

A remarkable restorative and rejuvenative herb with an affinity for the digestive and endocrine systems,

Glycyrrhiza glabra

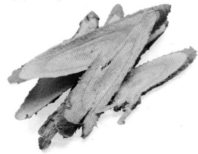

liquorice helps harmonize the qualities of other herbs, reducing heat, dryness and toxicity. It relieves acidity, heartburn and indigestion, colic, inflammatory problems and peptic ulcers. A mild laxative, it eases constipation. It increases bile flow from the liver and lowers cholesterol. It protects the liver from damage from toxins and infection.

An adaptogenic, strengthening tonic through its action on the adrenal glands, liquorice improves resilience to physical and mental stress. *Sattvic* in nature, it nourishes the brain, promotes good vision and memory, healthy hair and skin. It has anti-allergic effects similar to cortisone (but without the side-effects); it is useful when coming off orthodox steroids and for relieving hay fever, eczema, conjunctivitis and asthma.

A soothing expectorant, liquorice relieves irritation and inflammation in the chest, sore throats and dry coughs, bronchial congestion, asthma and chest infections. It enhances immunity and helps combat viruses, including *Cytomegalovirus* and *Herpes simplex*. It is good for convalescence and is anti-inflammatory for arthritis and skin problems, including eczema and psoriasis. It binds to toxic chemicals and carcinogens, and helps draw them from the body. Its mild oestrogenic properties help with both menstrual and menopausal problems.

Externally it may be used as a powder mixed with ghee, applied to wounds, herpes, eczema and psoriasis. A decoction with turmeric or Triphala can be used as a douche for thrush.

Cautions: Avoid prolonged use and large doses. Liquorice may increase fluid retention and blood pressure. Avoid during pregnancy. May cause potassium loss if combined with diuretics/laxatives. May potentiate Prednisolone.

Dosage: 3–5 gm powder daily.

Gymnema sylvestre
(Gurmar)

Part used: leaf
Quality: light, dry
Taste: bitter, astringent
Potency: cooling
Post-digestive: pungent
Dosha: PK- V+
Dhatu: plasma, blood, fat, reproductive
Srota: digestive, circulatory, urinary, reproductive

ACTIONS
Anti-diabetic, astringent, diuretic, laxative, refrigerant, lowers cholesterol, anti-obesity.

Gurmar is renowned for balancing blood sugar. Its Sanskrit name means 'sweet destroyer', because eating fresh leaves numbs bitter and sweet receptors on the tongue and reduces sweet cravings and excessive appetite. This is helpful for weight loss.

Gurmar helps the management of diabetes Types 1 and 2 and blood-sugar disorders. It increases the production of insulin by the pancreas, regulates blood glucose levels, stimulates the regeneration of beta cells in the pancreas that release insulin, and stops adrenaline from stimulating the liver to produce glucose. It also lowers cholesterol.

Cautions: It may aggravate gastro-oesophageal reflux. Avoid in hypoglycaemia and heart conditions. If taking hyperglycaemic drugs and insulin, monitor blood-sugar levels.

Dosage: 5–10 gm powder daily, 10–20 ml tincture daily

Hemidesmus indicus
(Sariva, Indian Sarsparilla)

Part used: bark of the root
Quality: light, oily
Taste: bitter, sweet, astringent
Potency: cooling
Post-digestive: sweet
Dosha: VPK=
Dhatu: blood, plasma, muscle,

reproductive, fat

Srota: digestive, circulatory, nerve, reproductive

ACTIONS

Digestive, laxative, depurative, anti-inflammatory, expectorant, antispasmodic, diuretic, febrifuge, fertility tonic, antihaemorrhagic, astringent, refrigerant, antimicrobial, diaphoretic, demulcent, antioxidant, aphrodisiac.

Sariva is a great cooling and cleansing remedy for excess *Pitta*. It is a *Rasayana* or rejuvenating tonic, as it has anabolic and strengthening properties. It increases the appetite and digestion, and is used for anorexia, indigestion, wind, bloating and diarrhoea. It clears *Ama* and dysbiosis and makes a good cleansing remedy for blood disorders, gout, arthritis and swollen glands.

It stimulates the flow of bile from the liver and supports the liver in its cleansing work. It enhances immunity and helps in auto-immune disease such as rheumatoid arthritis, psoriasis and lupus. It soothes inflammatory skin problems, including eczema, psoriasis, impetigo, scabies, herpes, ringworm and urticaria.

Sariva reduces *Pitta*-type fevers, including malarial fever. In hot water or mixed with honey, it reduces *Kapha* in the lungs, clear colds, catarrh, coughs, bronchitis and asthma.

It also relaxes tense muscles and calms the emotions. It balances all three *doshas* in the mind, particularly a disturbance of *Sadhaka Pitta* that causes irritability, intolerance, anger, criticism, self-criticism, PMS and depression.

Sariva balances the hormones, reduces heavy periods, improves fertility and helps prevent miscarriage. As an aphrodisiac, it improves sexual performance and sperm mobility. It also helps to prevent and treat anaemia. It purifies and increases breast milk, and is good for *Pitta*-type cystitis with burning, and for urinary stones and gravel.

Externally a paste applied to the skin reduces *Pitta*-type inflammation, swelling and burning. Sariva is also used in preparations for vaginal thrush. The fresh juice is used for conjunctivitis.

Dosage: 50–100 ml hot infusion daily, 3–6 gm powder daily

Hemidesmus indicus

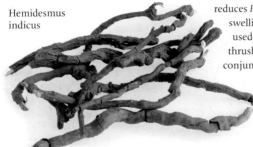

Momordica indica

(Karella/Karavella, Bitter Gourd)

Part used: whole plant
Quality: dry, light
Taste: bitter, pungent
Potency: hot
Post-digestive: pungent
Dosha: VKP=
Dhatu: plasma, blood, muscle, fat
Srota: digestive, urinary, excretory

ACTIONS

Antidiabetic, carminative, digestive, vermifuge, bitter tonic, diuretic, lithotriptic, alterative, vulnerary, anti-inflammatory, emmenagogue, galactogogue.

A very bitter vegetable resembling a cucumber, karella is excellent for reducing *Kapha* and lowering blood sugar. It is a good bitter tonic for anorexia, liver disorders, constipation, piles, gut infections, worms and parasites. It increases the absorption of nutrients and iron and combats anaemia. It clears toxins from the gut and excess acid via the urine. It is used for urinary stones and fluid retention. As a blood cleanser, it clears inflammatory skin conditions.

Externally the leaf juice is applied to skin problems and piles, and on the eyes in night-blindness.

Cautions: Avoid in pregnancy and in patients on hypoglycaemic medication.
Dosage: 60 ml daily of the fresh juice for diabetes, 5–10 gm dried daily, 3–15 ml tincture daily

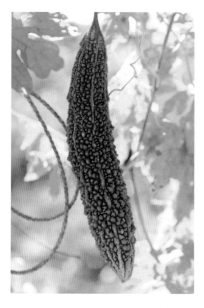

Momordica indica

Mucuna pruriens

(Kapikachu)

Part used: seed
Quality: heavy, unctuous
Taste: sweet, bitter
Potency: hot
Post-digestive: sweet
Dosha: VK- P=
Dhatu: all, especially nervous, reproductive
Srota: nervous, reproductive, respiratory

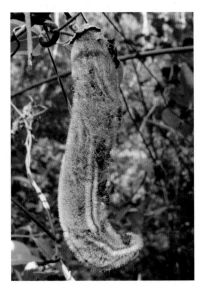

ACTIONS

Tonic, rejuvenative, astringent, anthelmintic, aphrodisiac, lowers blood sugar and prolactin, antihaemorrhagic, spermatogenic, hallucinogenic (in large doses), antispasmodic, antioxidant.

Famous as a remedy for Parkinson's disease, as the seeds contain L-dopa, kapikachu is a great tonic for the nerves, especially for *Vata* disorders. It is one of the best reproductive tonics and aphrodisiacs, used for low libido, impotence, low sperm count and infertility.

It is a good digestive and antispasmodic for intestinal pain and wind, spasm and constipation. The powder mixed with a teaspoon of ghee is useful in asthma and tight coughs.
Cautions: Avoid with *Ama* and congestion. Can irritate the gut and be overstimulating in excess. Often combined with milk and honey to increase its restorative effect.
Dosage: 3–10 gm powder two or three times daily, 3–15 ml tincture daily

Mucuna pruriens

Myristica fragrans

(Jati-phala, Nutmeg)

Part used: seed
Quality: light, oily penetrating
Taste: pungent, bitter, astringent
Potency: heating
Post-digestive: pungent
Dosha: VK- P+
Dhatu: plasma, muscle, bone, nerve, reproductive
Srota: digestive, nervous, excretory, reproductive

Myristica fragrans

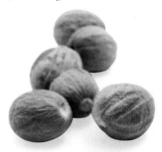

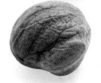

ACTIONS

Astringent, sedative, carminative, aphrodisiac, emmenagogue, circulatory stimulant, expectorant, digestive, liver tonic, anthelmintic, analgesic, anticonvulsant.

Nutmeg is excellent for calming *Vata* and a great aphrodisiac. It relieves convulsions, pain, insomnia, agitation, poor concentration, restless leg syndrome and arthritis. It is a reproductive tonic for infertility, low libido, impotence, irregular and painful periods. It helps prostate problems and incontinence.

This spice also enhances digestion and absorption, curbs diarrhoea and vomiting, spasms, wind and bloating. It relieves indigestion, liver disorders, colitis and worms. Warming and penetrating, it clears *Kapha* from the lungs and eases coughs, catarrh and rhinitis.

Externally it can be used as a paste/oil for headaches, arthritis and skin problems.

Cautions: Avoid with high *Pitta* and with sedatives, antihypertensives and antidepressants. Intoxicating in high doses (more than 6 gm).

Dosage: for sleep, 1/8 tsp in warm milk before bed, 0.5–6 gm or 1–6 ml tincture daily

Nigella sativa

(Kalonji/Krishna Jiraka, Black Cumin)

Part used: seeds
Quality: dry, light, penetrating
Taste: pungent, bitter
Potency: heating
Post-digestive: pungent
Dosha: VK- P+ (in excess)
Dhatu: plasma, blood, reproductive
Srota: digestive, urinary, female reproductive, excretory, respiratory

ACTIONS

Anti-allergenic, digestive, antispasmodic, liver tonic, depurative, hormone-balancing, nervine, galactagogue, anti-inflammatory.

These tasty seeds calm and strengthen the digestion, particularly when disturbed by *Vata*. They relieve wind, bloating, worms and parasites and aid fat metabolism. They clear excess *Kapha* from the lungs, relieving asthma, coughs and allergies such as hay fever.

A good brain tonic, kalonji calms the mind and enhances memory and concentration. It cleanses the liver, eases inflammatory eye disorders and *Pitta*-type headaches. It also reduces cysts and tumours, especially in the breast, clears *Kapha* from the uterus (as in fibroids and cysts) and reduces *Vata* symptoms, including painful and irregular periods. It also increases breast milk.

Externally the oil is applied for alopecia. It is used as *Nasya* in respiratory problems.

Cautions: Avoid in pregnancy.
Dosage: 1–10 gm powder daily, 3–12 ml tincture daily

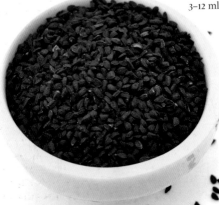

Nigella sativa

Ocimum sanctum

(Tulsi, Holy Basil)

Part used: leaves
Quality: light, sharp, dry
Taste: pungent, bitter
Potency: heating
Post-digestive: pungent
Dosha: VK- P+
Dhatu: plasma, blood, nerve, reproductive
Srota: respiratory, digestive, nervous, circulatory, urinary

ACTIONS

Demulcent, antimicrobial, expectorant, anticatarrhal, antispasmodic, probiotic, hypoglycaemic, anthelmintic, febrifuge, nervine, adaptogen, immunostimulant, digestive, laxative, antihistamine, hypotensive, diuretic.

One of the most sacred plants in India, tulsi has an uplifting and strengthening effect on mind and body. A wonderful adaptogen, it increases resilience to physical and emotional stress. It clears lethargy and congestion that dampen the spirits and fog the mind, and eases anxiety, depression, insomnia and stress-related problems, such as headaches, skin problems and IBS. It lowers blood sugar, cholesterol and triglyceride levels.

Decongestant, expectorant and antispasmodic, tulsi clears coughs, chest infections, colds, fevers, sore throats and flu, as well as histamine-induced allergies, including asthma and rhinitis. It is often used with ginger and black pepper for asthma. It helps combat microorganisms, including *E. coli*, *Staphylococcus aureus*, *Mycoplasma tuberculosis* and *Aspergillus*.

Antispasmodic and warming to the digestion, it improves appetite, digestion and absorption and relieves spasm and colic, wind and bloating. It is used for anorexia, nausea, vomiting, abdominal pain, constipation, peptic ulcers, irritation of the gut lining, infections, dysbiosis and worms.

Immune-enhancing and anti-inflammatory, tulsi protects healthy cells from toxicity caused by radiation and chemotherapy. It gives off ozone, an unstable form of oxygen that helps to break down chemicals and dispels disease-carrying organisms, such as viruses, bacteria and insects.

Tulsi helps to clear toxins through its diuretic effect and relieves painful urination, cystitis and urinary-tract infections.

Externally a juice of fresh leaves may be applied to skin conditions, including allergic rashes, athlete's foot and acne. Its antibiotic effect speeds healing.
Cautions: Avoid in pregnancy.
Dosage: 15–20 ml fresh juice with honey twice daily, 60–85 ml infusion thrice daily

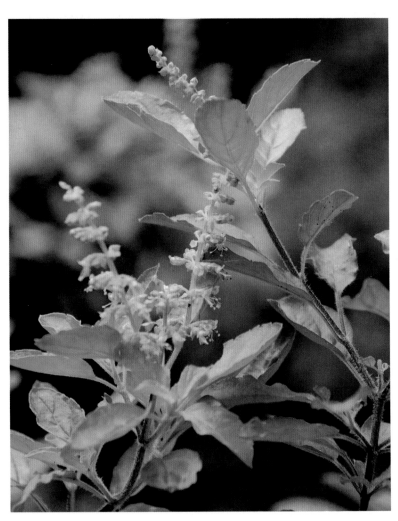

Ocimum sanctum

Phyllanthus amarus/niruri

(Bhumiamalaki, Phyllanthus, Stone Breaker)

Part used: leaves
Quality: dry, light
Taste: bitter, astringent, sweet
Potency: cooling
Post-digestive: sweet
Dosha: VPK=
Dhatu: plasma, blood, fat, bone, reproductive
Srota: digestive, reproductive, urinary, skeletal

ACTIONS

Antiviral, diuretic, alterative, cholagogue, laxative, antilithic, immunoregulator, haemostatic, hepatoprotective, digestive, anti-inflammatory, astringent, hypoglycaemic.

Cleansing for the liver and gall bladder, bhumiamalaki is a superb remedy for acute and chronic hepatitis and gall stones, and protects the liver from damage caused by chemicals, drugs and tobacco. It clears inflammatory skin problems, including eczema and urticaria. By calming *Pitta* it relieves hyperacidity, inflammatory gut problems, diarrhoea and dysentery, and clears heat and inflammation from the lower abdomen, reducing heavy bleeding and painful urination.

It helps dissolve urinary stones and gravel and regulates blood-sugar levels. It is excellent for lowered immunity, especially for viral conditions such as ME, HIV, flu and herpes.

Externally it is used for inflammatory skin and eye problems.

Cautions: Avoid in pregnancy.
Dosage: 1–6 mg leaves daily, 5–15 ml tincture daily

Piper longum

(Pippali, Long Pepper)

Part used: root, seeds
Quality: light, sharp, oily
Taste: pungent
Potency: heating
Post-digestive: sweet
Dosha: VK- P+
Dhatu: plasma, blood, fat, nerve, reproductive
Srota: circulatory, digestive, respiratory, reproductive

ACTIONS

Stimulant, carminative, laxative, diuretic, febrifuge, tonic, expectorant, anthelmintic, digestive, emollient, antiseptic, emmenagogue, rejuvenative, aphrodisiac, analgesic, cardiac stimulant.

Warming and energizing, pippali is an excellent tonic when you are cold and run-down, and the best *Rasayana* for *Kapha*. Used with ginger and black pepper in the famous formula Trikatu, it increases *Agni* and clears toxins in the gut and mucus in the lungs, enhancing the appetite, digestion and absorption by up to 30 per cent, and thereby increasing the effects of herbs and prescription drugs. It relieves anorexia, colic, wind, indigestion and constipation, combats amoeba, worms and candida, and enhances the liver's ability to break down toxins. It reduces liver damage from alcohol, drugs and chemicals.

Pippali stimulates the circulation, reduces harmful cholesterol and helps combat anaemia. It increases blood supply to the brain and calms *Vata*-related nervous problems, such as tension and spasm, restlessness, anxiety and insomnia; it also relieves stress-related problems such as headaches, constipation and IBS. It is a good warming and energizing reproductive tonic, it can be included in remedies for infertility and painful periods and it is reputed to be an aphrodisiac.

With its antimicrobial effects, pippali benefits the immune system, and is especially good for *Kapha* conditions, colds, catarrh, coughs, bronchitis, fevers, asthma and allergic conditions, including hay fever and eczema. Its antioxidant properties may explain its effects as a *Rasayana*. The root is used in gout, arthritis, muscle and back pain for its anti-inflammatory effects.

Externally it is used in liniments for pain and swelling, and is good as a mosquito repellent.

Cautions: Avoid in cases of acidity and during pregnancy. May increase drug absorption.

Dosage: 0.5–1 gm powdered seed and root in milk twice daily, as Trikatu 3 ml in hot water and honey 3 times daily before meals

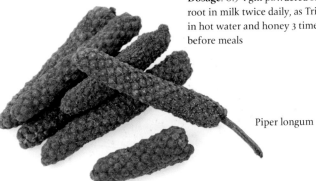

Piper longum

Plantago ovata

(Isaphogul, Psyllium Husk)

Part used: seeds, seed husk
Quality: unctuous, heavy, slimy
Taste: sweet
Potency: cool
Post-digestive: sweet
Dosha: VP- K+
Dhatu: plasma, blood, muscle
Srota: digestive, excretory, respiratory

ACTIONS

Laxative, demulcent, anti-inflammatory, anthelmintic, expectorant, emollient.

A demulcent bulk laxative, psyllium is excellent for constipation from dryness, as well as for diarrhoea, drawing toxins, mucus, bacteria, worms and amoeba from the gut, and helping to resolve inflammatory gut problems and dysbiosis. It soothes peptic ulcers and can reduce blood-sugar levels in Type 2 diabetes.

Its soluble fibre helps reduce harmful cholesterol. As a soothing demulcent, it eases dry *Vata*-type coughs and the pain and irritation in cystitis.

Externally it is anti-inflammatory and drawing, useful for headaches and boils.

Cautions: In excess it can dampen *Agni*, aggravate *Kapha* and *Ama*. Prolonged use may reduce fertility. Take two hours after other medication, as it may slow absorption. It may require changes to diabetic medication.

Dosage: 5–10 gm powder daily with plenty of liquid

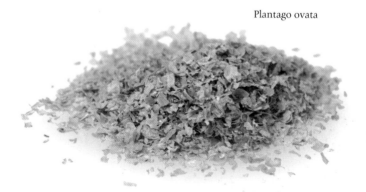

Plantago ovata

Plumbago zeylanicum

(Chitrak, White Leadwort)

Part used: root
Quality: dry, light, penetrating
Taste: pungent, bitter
Potency: very hot
Post-digestive: pungent
Dosha: VK- P +
Dhatu: plasma, blood, bone, reproductive
Srota: digestive, nerve, reproductive

ACTIONS

Stimulant, carminative, aphrodisiac, abortifacient, analgesic, rubefacient, anthelmintic, digestive, astringent, diaphoretic.

Hot and spicy, chitrak is a powerful heating remedy that stimulates *Agni* and clears toxins, promoting appetite, digestion and absorption as well as metabolism. It is superb for low digestive fire, anorexia, indigestion, colic, wind, bloating and diarrhoea, as well as liver disorders, piles and worms.

It moves stagnant *Vata* caused by a congestion of *Kapha*, and is excellent for nervous problems, arthritis with pain and fluid, and skin conditions, including vitiligo. It clears catarrh and coughs, rhinitis and fevers, and helps resolve menstrual and post-partum disorders and impotency.

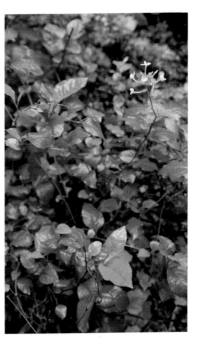

Plumbago zeylanicum

Externally it is rubefacient for arthritis and skin problems, including vitiligo. It may cause blistering.
Cautions: Avoid in pregnancy, high *Pitta*. Use sparingly with other herbs, ghee or lime juice; an overdose can cause burning, vomiting and diarrhoea.
Dosage: 250 mg–3 gm powder, 1–6 ml tincture

Pueraria tuberosa

(Vidari Kanda)

Part used: tuber
Quality: heavy, unctuous
Taste: sweet
Potency: cold
Post-digestive: sweet
Dosha: PV- K+
Dhatu: plasma, blood, muscle, fat, reproductive
Srota: reproductive, nervous, digestive

ACTIONS

Diuretic, nutritive tonic, anabolic, galactagogue, cholagogue, alterative, carminative, cardiotonic, haemostatic, demulcent, aphrodisiac, rejuvenative.

A relative of the sweet potato, vidari is sweet, moistening and nourishing. It is a renowned rejuvenating tonic for *Vata* and the reproductive system, and especially good for nervous exhaustion, debility, underweight, convalescence and old age. It increases sperm production, sexual energy and performance and enhances fertility. It reduces heavy periods, strengthens women after childbirth and increases breast milk, as it nourishes *Rasa dhatu* and the channels that carry breast milk.

Vidari balances *Vata* and *Pitta* in the lower abdomen and clears inflammation and dryness from the digestive tract; it is helpful in constipation and conditions of the urinary tract, soothing pain and cystitis. It eases sore throats, hoarseness, coughs and catarrh.

Dosage: 1–15 gm powder daily, 3–15 ml tincture daily

Rubia cordifolia

(Manjishta, Indian Madder)

Part used: root
Quality: heavy, dry
Taste: sweet, bitter, astringent
Potency: hot
Post-digestive: pungent
Dosha: PK- V+
Dhatu: plasma, blood, nerves, muscles
Srota: circulatory, reproductive, bone, nervous, excretory

ACTIONS

Alterative, diuretic, emmenagogue, astringent, febrifuge, antitumour, haemostatic, rejuvenative, anti-inflammatory, antioxidant, hepatoprotective, digestive.

One of the best *Pitta*-reducing, detoxifying herbs, manjishta clears heat and *Ama* from the blood and is a good remedy for fevers and inflammatory conditions. It is excellent for stubborn skin problems, reducing heat and itching in eczema, psoriasis, herpes, acne, scabies and athlete's foot, and when taken with honey it is used for vitiligo. It is also one of the main herbs for stopping bleeding, as in heavy periods, nosebleeds, bleeding ulcers and inflammatory gut problems.

Manjishta enhances immunity and has been used to relieve inflammatory chest problems and infections, including tuberculosis, allergic asthma, arthritis and auto-immune problems. Greatly beneficial to the liver, manjishta protects it against damage from infections and toxins and is used for hepatitis. With its antioxidant properties it has a reputation as a rejuvenative.

Manjishta improves the appetite and clears toxins from the gut, and is good for diarrhoea with bleeding, Crohn's disease, worms and dysentery. It eases nervous disorders associated with excess *Pitta*, such as irritability, intolerance, anger, depression and low self-esteem.

It has the ability to break up accumulations of *Kapha* in the bladder, liver and kidneys, including urinary stones and gravel. It also helps urinary-tract infections, blood in the urine, painful and irregular periods and endometriosis related to excess *Pitta* and *Kapha*. It is used to prevent miscarriage and purifies breast milk.

Externally it stops bleeding and speeds the healing of cuts and wounds. It also eases inflammatory eye problems. The paste mixed with honey is used for inflammatory skin problems and ulcers.

Cautions: Avoid with high *Vata*.
Dosage: 1–3 gm powder daily, 60–120 ml decoction daily

Rubia cordifolia

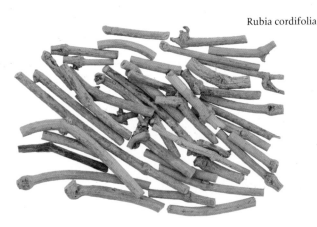

Saraca indica

(Ashoka)

Part used: bark
Quality: light, dry
Taste: bitter, astringent
Potency: cold
Post-digestive: pungent
Dosha: KP- V+
Dhatu: blood, muscle, fat, reproductive
Srota: female reproductive, circulatory

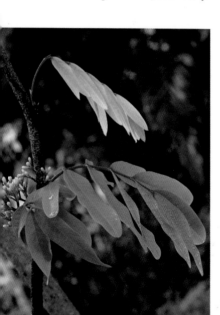

ACTIONS

Astringent, uterine tonic, alterative, analgesic, diuretic, cardio-tonic, anthelmintic, haemostatic, antispasmodic, nervine.

Ashoka is an excellent tonic for the uterus, particularly for reducing heavy bleeding. By strengthening the uterine muscles and clearing congestion, it is good for prolapse, painful and irregular periods, fibroids, cysts and endometriosis. It helps prevent miscarriage.

It is good for *Vata*-type nervous problems, calming anxiety, restlessness and relieving pain and insomnia. It tones the lining of the gut, protecting it from irritation and infection. It relieves indigestion, gastritis, colitis, peptic ulcers, bleeding piles, diarrhoea, dysentery and worms. As a diuretic, it reduces fluid retention, relieves cystitis and helps prevent the formation of stones and gravel.

Externally it is applied to relieve nerve pain.

Cautions: Avoid in cases of constipation.
Dosage: 1–9 gm powder daily, 3–15 ml tincture daily

Saraca indica

Sida cordifolia

(Bala, Indian Country Mallow)

Part used: root, leaves
Quality: unctuous, heavy
Taste: bitter, sweet
Potency: sweet
Post-digestive: cooling
Dosha: VPK= K+ (in excess)
Dhatu: all, especially nerve
Srota: nervous, reproductive, circulatory, urinary, respiratory

ACTIONS
Astringent, stomachic, tonic, febrifuge, demulcent, diuretic, antispasmodic, analgesic, antimicrobial, adaptogenic, rejuvenative, nervine.

A great tonic and rejuvenative, bala is one of the best adaptogenic and nourishing herbs for *Vata*, increasing *Ojas*, enhancing energy, vitality, immunity, fertility and resilience to stress. In fact bala literally means 'strength'. It relieves tension, anxiety, nervous exhaustion and insomnia, as well as headaches, shingles, and nerve, muscle and joint pain.

Bala eases dry coughs, asthma and chronic infections related to debility, including bronchitis, bronchiectasis and ME. It soothes inflammatory gut problems, including gastritis, acidity, colitis, IBS, colic and wind, and relieves urinary-tract infections.

Externally it is used as an oil for muscle and nerve pain, arthritis and eye disorders.
Cautions: It contains ephedrine and may interact with MAO inhibitors, steroids and beta-blockers.
Dosage: 1–3 gm in a milk decoction 2–3 times daily

Terminalia belerica

(Bibhitaki, Beleric Myrobalan)

Part used: fruit
Quality: light, dry
Taste: sweet, astringent
Potency: heating
Post-digestive: sweet
Dosha: VPK= V+ (in excess)
Dhatu: plasma, muscle, bone, nerve
Srota: respiratory, digestive, excretory, nervous

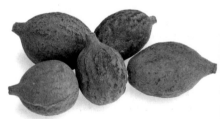

Terminalia belerica

ACTIONS

Laxative, expectorant, bronchodilator, nervine, antimicrobial, tonic, immunostimulant, anti-inflammatory, astringent, anthelmintic, lithotrophic, antioxidant, rejuvenative, antihistamine.

An excellent rejuvenative for *Kapha* and the lungs, bibhitaki enhances immunity and when taken as a powder with honey can relieve coughs, colds, sore throats and catarrh as well as allergies, including eczema, asthma and rhinitis.

It cleanses and regulates the bowels and is included in prescription for haemorrhoids, worms and both diarrhoea and constipation. It soothes inflammatory bowel problems such as colitis, Crohn's disease and ulcers, and forms one-third of the famous formula Triphala. Bibhitaki protects the liver and can be used to treat liver problems and gall stones. Although it is heating it does not aggravate *Pitta*.

Bibhitaki makes a good brain tonic, especially for *Vata problems*, including insomnia. It helps arthritis, lowers cholesterol and removes *Kapha* accumulations in the urinary tract that cause stones and gravel.

Externally it speeds the healing of wounds. It is also used in hair oils and for skin problems. The powder can be mixed with a little water and used as a gargle for sore throats and impaired voice.

Dosage: 2 gm powder twice daily

Terminalia chebula

(Haritaki, Indian Gall Nut)

Part used: fruit, leaves, stem, bark
Quality: light, dry
Taste: mainly bitter and astringent; also sour, pungent, sweet
Potency: heating
Post-digestive: sweet
Dosha: tridosha
Dhatu: all
Srota: respiratory, digestive, excretory, nervous

ACTIONS

Tonic, anti-inflammatory, laxative, astringent, antiseptic, diuretic, alterative, carminative, demulcent, febrifuge, bronchodilator, anthelmintic, cardiotonic, vulnerary, hypotensive, antioxidant, adaptogenic, rejuvenative.

An excellent antioxidant, nerve and brain tonic, haritaki enhances resilience to stress, promotes intellect and sight, improves longevity and is recommended for all *Vata* disorders. It protects the heart and arteries from damage by free radicals, reduces blood pressure and lowers harmful cholesterol, thereby helping to slow the ageing process and living up to its reputation as a rejuvenative.

By increasing *Agni* it promotes the appetite, digestion and absorption, corrects the flow of *Apana Vata* and

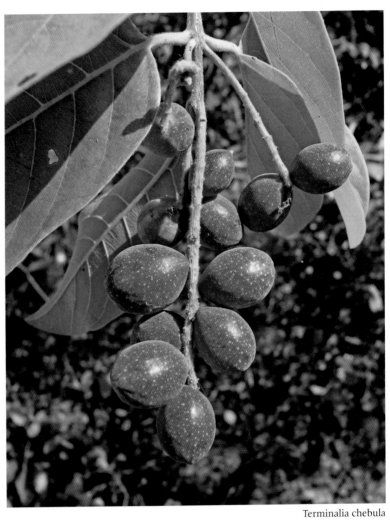

Terminalia chebula

regulates the bowels, correcting either constipation or diarrhoea, according to the dosage. It is excellent for all *Vata* digestive problems and alleviates indigestion, colic, wind, constipation, haemorrhoids, IBS, diarrhoea and vomiting. It can also be used for infections such as *Shigella* spp. and *Salmonella typhi* and for parasites including amoebas, as well as for inflammation of the mucous membranes and ulcers. The unripe fruits are more laxative than the ripe ones, which are more astringent.

Haritaki enhances immunity and helps combat bacterial and viral infections. It can be used for urinary-tract infections and cystitis, candida and *Cytomegalovirus* and may have antitumour activity. Its astringent properties help in prolapse and to reduce excessive discharges, including catarrh, *Kapha*-type mucousy coughs, sweating and menorrhagia. It relieves fevers and asthma, purifies breast milk and clears skin problems.

Externally haritaki can be used as a gargle and mouthwash for mouth ulcers, bleeding/infected gums and sore throats.
Cautions: Avoid in pregnancy, dehydration, emaciation, high *Pitta*.
Dosage: 3–6 gm powder daily as a laxative, 1 gm powder daily as a *Rasayana*, 55–110 ml decoction daily; for a laxative effect use with warm water; for an astringent effect use with cold water

Tinospora cordifolia
(Guduchi, Amrit)

Part used: stem, root
Quality: light, oily
Taste: bitter, astringent, pungent, sweet
Potency: hot
Post-digestive: sweet
Dosha: VPK=
Dhatu: plasma, blood, muscle, nerve, fat, reproductive
Srota: circulatory, digestive

ACTIONS
Digestive, astringent, rejuvenative, nervine, tonic, alterative, antimicrobial, febrifuge, diuretic, antioxidant, adaptogen, hepato-protective, cholagogue, anti-inflammatory, probiotic.

An excellent *Rasayana*, especially for *Pitta*, guduchi enhances immunity, longevity, energy and vitality. It helps fight off infection, increases resilience to emotional and physical stress, promotes brain function and eases tension. By enhancing immunity guduchi relieves acute respiratory infections, fevers, coughs, colds, flu, sinusitis and allergies, including hay fever and asthma. Taken prior to surgery, it helps prevent post-operative complications including infections. It has antioxidant and

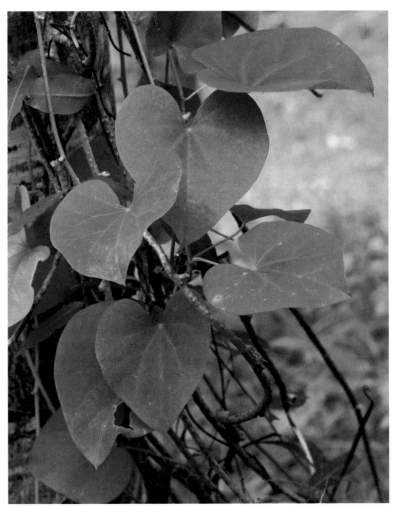

Tinospora cordifolia

anti-tumour activity and protects against the toxic effects of chemotherapy and radiotherapy.

Guduchi improves digestion, absorption and liver function, promotes gut flora and clears *Ama* from the gut and *srotas*, particularly the brain. It promotes metabolism of all tissues, especially fat, helping regulate weight. By reducing heat and inflammation, guduchi soothes acidity, gastritis, peptic ulcers, diarrhoea, gut infections, nausea and vomiting. It is used with ghee for constipation. It protects the liver against damage from toxins, drugs and alcohol, aids liver regeneration and is used for chronic hepatitis. It clears heat, toxins and uric acid by increasing urination, and relieves inflammatory and auto-immune disease, including rheumatoid arthritis, psoriasis and lupus. It eases gout (in castor oil) and arthritis (with ginger).

It is also good for *Pitta* problems, including anaemia and bleeding (as in bleeding gums and haemorrhoids). It reduces cholesterol and helps to stabilize blood-sugar levels. It is used for obstinate inflammatory skin problems such as eczema, and as a reproductive tonic for impotence and sexual debility.

Externally, as a powder mixed with water or aloe-vera gel, it is applied to inflammatory skin problems.

Cautions: Avoid in pregnancy.

Dosage: 3–5 gm powder twice daily

Tribulus terrestris
(Gokshura, Caltrops)

Part used: fruit
Quality: heavy, oily
Taste: sweet, bitter
Potency: cooling
Post-digestive: sweet
Dosha: VPK=
Dhatu: plasma, blood, nerve, reproductive
Srota: urinary, reproductive, nervous, respiratory

ACTIONS
Diuretic, lithotriptic, digestive, astringent, anthelmintic, laxative, demulcent, cardiotonic, rejuvenative, aphrodisiac, nervine, analgesic.

An excellent *Rasayana* for *Pitta* and *Vata*, gokshura increases *Sattva*, promotes clarity, calms the nerves and relieves pain. It is traditionally taken with equal amounts of dry ginger for nerve and back pain.

It is an excellent energy tonic when taken with ashwagandha, enhancing resilience to stress and improving energy and sports performance.

Taken in a milk decoction, it acts as an aphrodisiac. It strengthens the reproductive tract, and is used for infertility, low libido, impotency and prostate problems. It also helps prevent miscarriage and speeds recovery after childbirth.

A rejuvenating kidney tonic and soothing diuretic, gokshura relieves oedema, cystitis, haematuria, urinary-tract infections and incontinence. It enhances the elimination of toxins, stones and gravel, and relieves gout, arthritis and sciatica. It improves cardiac circulation, reduces blood pressure and is a good expectorant for coughs and asthma.

Externally the oil is used for alopecia and premature balding.

Cautions: Avoid in pregnancy.
Dosage: 2–5 gm powder daily, 60–100 ml milk or water decoction daily

Tribulus terrestris

Trigonella foenum-graecum

(Methi, Fenugreek)

Part used: seeds; leaves used as a vegetable or salad
Quality: light, oily
Taste: pungent, astringent, sweet, bitter
Potency: hot
Post-digestive: pungent
Dosha: VK- P+
Dhatu: plasma, blood, fat, nerve, reproductive
Srota: digestive, excretory, respiratory, reproductive

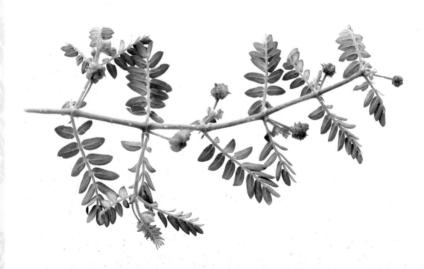

ACTIONS

Digestive, laxative, demulcent, nutritive, galactogogue, expectorant, antimicrobial, antihypertensive, hypoglycaemic, lowers cholesterol, rejuvenative, aphrodisiac, diuretic.

Highly nutritious, fenugreek aids digestion and makes a good tonic for convalescence and debility. Its mucilaginous fibre soothes gastritis, acidity and peptic ulcers. It acts as a bulk laxative for constipation. It inhibits carbohydrate and cholesterol absorption and dissolves fat, reduces blood pressure and clotting, helping to prevent cardiovascular disease and diabetes.

Fenugreek increases libido and reduces menopausal symptoms. It can enlarge the breasts and stimulates milk flow. It is an expectorant for coughs, and antiviral for colds and flu. As a diuretic, it aids the elimination of toxins.

Externally it is used for skin problems and mouth ulcers.

Cautions: Avoid in pregnancy, and with antidiabetic and anticoagulant drugs.

Dosage: 1–3 gm powder twice daily

Valeriana wallichi

(Tagarah, Indian Valerian)

Part used: roots
Quality: light, oily
Taste: bitter, pungent, astringent, sweet
Potency: heating
Post-digestive: pungent
Dosha: VPK=
Dhatu: plasma, blood, muscle, nerve
Srota: digestive, respiratory, nervous

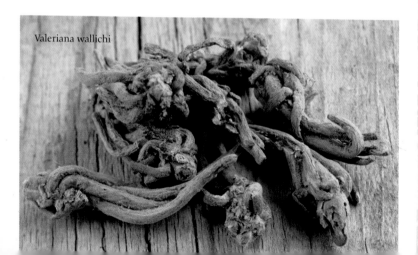

Valeriana wallichi

ACTIONS

Antispasmodic, nervine, hypotensive, carminative, digestive, cardiostimulant, laxative, hepatostimulant.

Warming and grounding, tagarah is excellent for anxiety, tension, panic attacks, agitation, hysteria and when taken before bed for insomnia. A good alternative to orthodox sedatives, it helps withdrawal from drugs and cigarettes. As an aid to memory and concentration, it is helpful in ADHD.

Tagarah can be used for stress-related heart and blood-pressure problems, including palpitations. It enhances digestion, regulates *Apana Vata* and eases *Vata*-related muscle tension and cramps, constipation, pain, wind, bloating and period pain. It clears catarrh and helps asthma and tight coughs.

Externally a paste may be applied to headaches, on wounds, fractures and arthritis to speed healing.

Cautions: Avoid in pregnancy, high *Pitta* and with antihypertensives.

Dosage: 1–3 gm powder daily

Vitex negundo

(Nirgundi, Chaste Tree)

Part used: whole plant
Quality: light, dry
Taste: bitter, pungent, astringent
Potency: heating
Post-digestive: hot
Dosha: VK- P+ (in excess)
Dhatu: blood, nerve, bone, reproductive
Srota: reproductive, digestive, nervous

ACTIONS

Astringent, analgesic, anti-inflammatory, hepatoprotective, anti-allergenic, antibacterial, vulnerary, nervine, antispasmodic, sedative, rejuvenative.

Excellent for *Vata*, nirgundi nourishes the brain and nerves, eases pain and relieves headaches, sciatica, arthritis, PMS, poor memory and concentration. It helps drug withdrawal and eases muscle spasms and menstrual cramps.

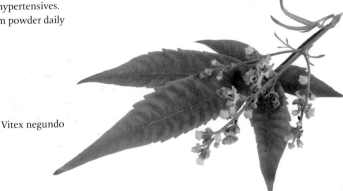

Vitex negundo

By increasing *Agni* and clearing *Ama* nirgundi improves digestion and absorption. It relieves indigestion, wind, dysbiosis, worms and hepatitis. It reduces fevers, inflammation and skin problems. By clearing *Kapha* from the lungs it helps catarrh, coughs and asthma. As a diuretic it eases cystitis and oedema.

Externally it is used for cleaning wounds, conjunctivitis, bruises, sprains, skin problems, headaches and mouth ulcers; and as an oil for arthritis, as a hair tonic and for ear infections.

Cautions: Avoid with sedative/antidepressant drugs, contraceptives and HRT.

Dosage: 10–12 ml leaf juice daily, 1–3 gm powder daily

Withania somniferum

(Ashwagandha, Winter Cherry)

Part used: root
Quality: light, oily
Taste: sweet, bitter, pungent
Potency: hot
Post-digestive: sweet
Dosha: VK- P+
Dhatu: blood, muscle, fat, bone, nerve, reproductive
Srota: reproductive, nervous, respiratory

ACTIONS

Sedative, nervine, nutritive, rejuvenative, anti-inflammatory, adaptogenic, antioxidant, tonic, aphrodisiac, astringent, antispasmodic, anticonvulsant, diuretic, cardioprotective, hypotensive, thyroid stimulant, immunomodulatory.

Ashwagandha is an exceptional nourishing nerve tonic and *Rasayana*, especially for *Vata*. It promotes energy, strength and vitality and is recommended during convalescence, for weakness and emaciation, and for problems of old age, including poor memory, weak eyes, arthritis and insomnia. Its antioxidant properties limit damage from free radicals and reduce ageing.

Ashwagandha improves resilience to physical and emotional stress, and is excellent when run-down by chronic illness, stress, anxiety, overwork, panic attacks, nervous exhaustion or insomnia. It is *Sattvic*, engendering calmness, wisdom and clarity, and helps children with behavioural problems and ADHD.

Ashwagandha enhances immunity and may help prevent and treat cancer, increasing the sensitivity of cancer cells to radiation therapy and making it more effective. A good painkiller and anti-inflammatory for joint problems, it can help auto-immune problems, including MS, psoriasis, ankylosing

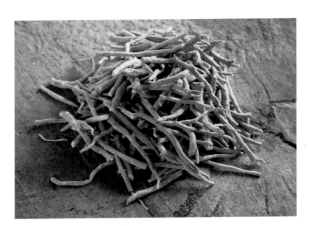

Withania
somniferum

spondylitis and rheumatoid arthritis.
Ashwagandha increases resistance to
respiratory infections and is used for
allergies, rhinitis and asthma due to
aggravated *Vata*.

Ashwagandha is the best regulator of
Apana Vata, which governs the lower
abdomen. It is excellent for urinary
problems, painful periods and menstrual
problems associated with excess *Vata*,
including irregular and scanty periods
and endometriosis. It is famous for
infertility and as a male reproductive
tonic.

Externally the oil is used for painful
joints, frozen shoulder, nerve pain such
as sciatica, numbness, muscle spasm and
back pain. It heals wounds, sores and
dry, itchy skin conditions, such as eczema
and psoriasis.

Cautions: Avoid in pregnancy, excess
Pitta.
Dosage: 5 gm powder in warm water or
milk twice daily

Zingiber officinale

(Adrak [fresh], Sunthi [dried], Ginger)

Part used: rhizomes
Quality: light, oily
Taste: pungent
Potency: heating
Post-digestive: sweet
Dosha: VK- P+
Dhatu: all
Srota: digestive, respiratory, circulatory

ACTIONS

Thermogenic, peripheral circulatory stimulant, carminative, laxative, digestive, expectorant, diuretic, aphrodisiac, laxative, anti-emetic, analgesic, anthelmintic, anti-inflammatory, antiplatelet, antioxidant, diaphoretic.

Pungent and warming, ginger is a wonderful aid to digestion, excellent for nausea from travel sickness, pregnancy, overeating, anxiety and infection. It increases the appetite, is useful in anorexia, and clears toxins and dysbiosis, increasing health and vitality and enhancing immunity. It is good for IBS and food allergies. Pain-relieving and relaxing, it also relieves colic and spasm, wind and bloating, and griping from diarrhoea and dysentery.

Ginger enhances immunity and combats bacterial and viral infections, such as gut infections, colds and flu,

Zingiber officinale

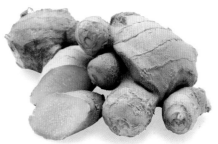

acute and chronic bronchitis. It is excellent when taken hot at the onset of respiratory infections. It clears fevers, colds, catarrh, headaches, coughs, chest infections, bronchitis, bronchietasis and asthma.

Ginger is *Sattvic* and rejuvenating. As an antioxidant it protects against the ageing process. It stimulates the heart and circulation, creating a feeling of warmth and well-being and restoring vitality. It reduces blood-clotting and helps dizziness, poor circulation, chilblains and Raynaud's disease. With its anti-inflammatory and detoxifying properties, it also eases osteoarthritis and rheumatoid arthritis.

As a reproductive tonic, ginger has aphrodisiac effects, being excellent for impotence caused by a deficiency of warmth. It regulates the flow of *Apana Vata* and relieves delayed, painful and scanty periods and clots.

Externally you can chew fresh ginger to relieve toothache, and use grated or powdered ginger as a paste to cover the scalp to promote hair growth. In oils it is useful for lumbago, neuralgia and painful joints aggravated by cold.

Cautions: Avoid with peptic ulcers, gall stones and high *Pitta*. Avoid with anticoagulants.

Dosage: 2–5 gm fresh ginger or 2–10 ml tincture daily, 1–2 gm dried ginger or 1–2 ml tincture daily

Chapter 16: **Traditional preparations and formulae**

Ayurvedic herbs are traditionally prepared in a wide variety of different ways. There are many advantages to using preparations and formulae. They enable many herbs to be used together in one prescription, enhance the digestion and absorption of the remedy, augment its potency and effect, and are a means of preserving the herbs so that they do not deteriorate quickly.

Certain preparations are indicated for particular diseases or are suited to specific plants. They are generally available through Ayurvedic suppliers, and from India and Sri Lanka. If you prefer, you can formulate your own prescriptions according to your individual needs.

The main herbal preparations and formulae (*Bheshajya kalpana*) are described in this chapter.

Dried and fresh herbs can be prepared in many different ways to suit the needs of each person.

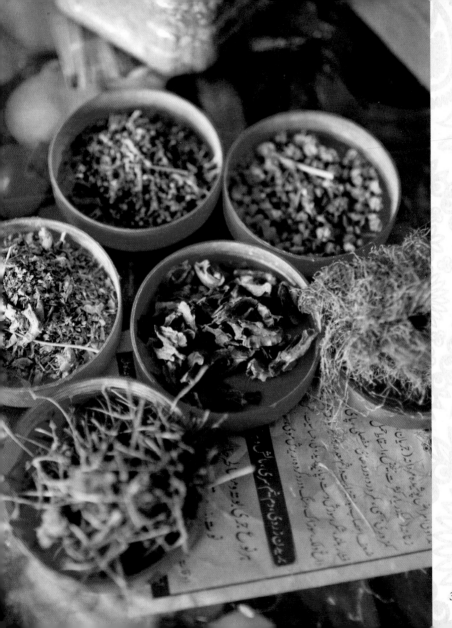

Herbal powders (*Churnas*)

Dried plants are ground into powders which can be made into tablets to prolong their shelf life, as they tend to deteriorate quickly. There are many famous *Churnas*, including Triphala and Trikatu. They are generally taken as ½–1 teaspoon in milk, water or honey, depending on the vehicle suited to the *dosha* being treated.

Avipattikar Churna

Ingredients: dry ginger, black pepper, long pepper, haritaki, bibhitaki, amalaki, musta, bidam, cardamom, bay leaves, cloves, trivrut and sharkara (sugar)

Properties: carminative, antacid, laxative, cholagogue, anti-emetic, nervine

Uses: a wonderful remedy to clear excess *Vata*, *Pitta* and *Ama*. A good laxative for *Pitta* aggravation, *Avipattikar* clears inflammatory acids and toxins from the system, balances the digestive fire, cools hyperacidity and heartburn, redirects the flow of *Apana Vata* downward, helps *Pitta*-type

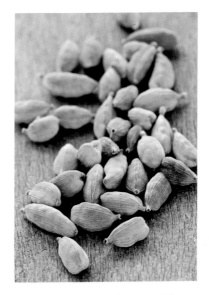

Cardamom seeds are used in many different formulae for aiding digestion.

headaches and relieves skin problems.
Dosage: 2–5 gm three times a day with warm water, to prevent griping from aggravated *Vata*
Caution: avoid in pregnancy

Dashmoola
(10 Roots)
Ingredients: kantakari, bruhati, shaliparni, pushniparni, gokshura, bilwa, shyonaka, patala, kashmari and agnimantha
Properties: expectorant, anti-asthmatic, nervine, febrifuge, analgesic
Uses: an excellent anti-inflammatory, digestive, tonic, nervine, relaxant, analgesic and anti-arthritic combination, making it a superb choice for *Vata* aggravations; for spasms, tremors, lumbago, sciatica, arthritis, nerve pain, debility, stroke paralysis, tinnitus, anxiety, fear, depression and old age. Traditionally *Dashmoola* is also used for herbal enemas.
Dosage: 50 ml (2 fl oz) of the decoction twice a day with long-pepper powder

Hingwashtaka Churna
(Asafoetida 8 Compound)
Ingredients: asafoetida, ginger, black pepper, long pepper, rock salt, cumin, black cumin, ajwan
Properties: carminative, stimulant, antispasmodic; decreases *Vata* and *Kapha*, increases *Pitta*
Uses: abdominal distension, wind, colic, indigestion, dysbiosis, infection
Dosage: 1–4 gm or 2–8 tablets two to three times daily in warm water

Lavanbhaskar Churna
(Five-Salts Compound)
Ingredients: 5 salts (rock salt, black salt, sea salt, sambhar salt, ammonium chloride), fennel, long pepper, long-pepper root, black cumin, cinnamon leaf, nagakeshar, talisha, rhubarb root, pomegranate seeds, cinnamon, cardamom

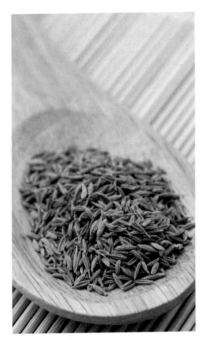

Cumin is an excellent spice for the digestion. It enhances absorption and metabolism and clears toxins from the gut.

Lavangadi

Ingredients: cloves, camphor, cardamom, cinnamon, nutmeg, vetiver, ginger, cumin, bamboo manna, jatamansi, long pepper, sandalwood, cubeb, raw sugar

Properties: carminative, digestive, antimicrobial, decongestant. Reduces *Vata* and *Kapha*, and increases *Agni* and *Pitta*; clears *Ama*.

Uses: poor appetite, colds, coughs, gas, colic, diarrhoea, nausea and vomiting

Dosage: 2–5 gm before meals in warm water

Properties: stimulant, carminative, laxative. Decreases *Vata*, increases *Agni* and *Pitta*

Uses: loss of appetite, malabsorption, constipation, abdominal pain

Dosage: 1–4 gm or 2–8 tablets two to three times daily in warm water or buttermilk

Mahasudarshan Churna

Ingredients: bitters including chiretta, guduchi, barberry, ginger, long pepper, black pepper, Triphala

Properties: febrifuge, antimicrobial, bitter tonic, diaphoretic, diuretic, alterative. Reduces *Pitta* and *Ama*.

Uses: excellent cleansing remedy

for the prevention and treatment of flu, fevers, debility after fevers, nausea, enlargement of the liver and spleen. Mainly anti-*Pitta*, it helps the liver in its detoxifying work after exposure to toxic chemicals or eating allergenic foods. It can be used for acne, boils and rashes, and is excellent during the allergy season. It is recommended for people who are sensitive to chemicals or with multiple food allergies. Half a teaspoon taken before breakfast with a little honey relieves cravings for sugar or carbohydrates in high-*Pitta* people. **Dosage**: 1–4 gm or 2–8 tablets two to three times daily in water

Rasayana Churna
Ingredients: guduchi, gokshura, amalaki
Properties: bitter tonic, demulcent, alterative, diuretic, antacid
Uses: general debility, sexual debility, skin rashes, allergies, chronic fevers or infections. A good rejuvenative tonic for *Pitta*, particularly after febrile diseases.
Dosage: 1–4 gm or 2–8 tablets two to three times daily in raw sugar and ghee, or in milk

Sitopaladi Churna
Ingredients: rock candy, bamboo manna, long pepper, cardamom, cinnamon
Properties: expectorant, antitussive, decongestant;

Half a teaspoon of Sitopaladi Churna *in a little honey or water is a great decongestant.*

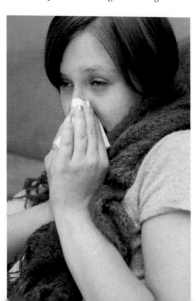

increases *Agni*.
Uses: colds, coughs, lack of appetite, fever, debility. A major anti-*Kapha* formula, which reduces *Vata*.
Dosage: 1–4 gm or 2–8 tablets two to four times daily in honey or ghee

Talisadi Churna

Ingredients: talisha, Trikatu, bamboo manna, cardamom, cinnamon, raw sugar
Properties: expectorant, antitussive, stimulant, decongestant. Increases *Agni* in *Vata* and *Kapha* conditions.
Uses: colds, flu, bronchitis, loss of appetite, indigestion, chronic fever; mainly anti-*Kapha*
Dosage: 1–4 gm or 2–8 tablets twice daily in honey or lime juice

Trikatu Churna

Ingredients: black pepper, long pepper, ginger
Properties: stimulant, expectorant, decongestant, digestive. Increases *Agni*, clears *Ama*. Reduces *Kapha* and *Vata*, increases *Pitta*.
Uses: lack of appetite, indigestion, cough, congestion. Specific for low *Agni* and high *Ama*
Dosage: 1–3 gm or 2–6 tablets two to three times daily in honey or warm water

Triphala Churna

(Three Fruits)
Ingredients: the fruit of three tropical trees called 'myrobalan plums' – haritaki, amalaki and bibhitaki – each one balancing one of the three *doshas*
Properties: laxative, tonic, rejuvenative, astringent, alterative, antioxidant, probiotic, antimicrobial, eye tonic. Good for all three *doshas*.
Uses: chronic constipation, wind and bloating, eye problems, chronic diarrhoea. The most famous Ayurvedic compound, Triphala is considered the best and safest bowel-cleanser, as well as a tonic and rejuvenative (*Rasayana*). It improves digestive

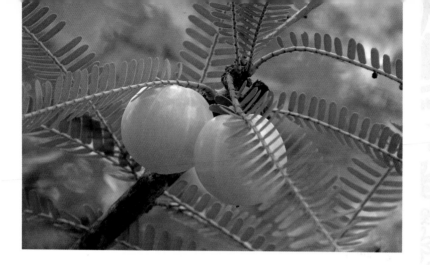

fire, enhancing appetite and digestion, and has a reputation for nourishing the nervous system. It is good for constipation in any of the *doshas*, although it is not always effective in acute constipation. As a metabolic regulator it helps to reduce weight, while having a strengthening and nutritive effect upon deeper tissues, including blood, muscle and nerve tissue in those who are underweight. It reduces cholesterol, protects the heart, reduces raised blood pressure, improves liver function and has anti-inflammatory and antiviral properties.

Amalaki is one of the ingredients of Triphala and is famous as one of the best healing and rejuvenative remedies of Ayurveda.

Triphala can be taken with digestive spices such as Trikatu, thus combining a bowel-cleanser (*Ama pachana*) with remedies to raise the digestive fire (*Agni deepana*). It is useful not only in *Ama* conditions, but as part of a regular diet for preventing the accumulation of *Ama*.

Dosage: 5–10 gm once daily in warm water, ghee or honey before sleep.

Other herbal preparations

There are many other forms of herbal preparation, including decoctions and infusions, herbal jams and jellies, juices and pastes, wines and tinctures, gugguls (pills) and medicated ghees and oils.

Decoctions

A decoction (*Kvatha*) is made by adding one part of dry herb to 16 parts of water, then reducing it to four parts of the original volume of water (or you can halve the proportions ½:8:2) by simmering. Roots, bark, stems and fruit are usually decocted.

For milk decoctions (*Ksirapaka kalpana*) one part of herb is mixed with eight parts of milk and 32 parts of water and simmered until the water evaporates. This is generally recommended for *Rasayana* treatments (such as *Pippali vardhaman*, where increasing numbers of long-pepper fruits are taken to treat asthma) as well as for lipid-soluble components, such as saponins.

Herbal stocks (*Panaka*) are made by simmering one part of herb in 64 parts of water and then reducing it to half. Rice or vegetable soups are then made in this stock as a part of *Rasayana* therapy.

Hot infusions (*Phantha*)

The softer parts of a plant – the leaves, stems and flowers – are usually made into infusions. One part of herb is infused in a pot in eight parts of freshly boiled water. This brew is left to steep for up to 12 hours and is taken hot for *Vata* and *Kapha* problems.

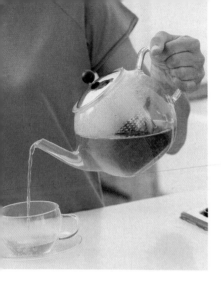

Herbal infusions are taken hot for Vata and Kapha problems.

left overnight, when the cooling lunar energy is at its peak. Well-known preparations are made from guduchi, coriander seed (see below), fennel seed and raisins, jasmine flowers and sariva.

Herbal jams, jellies, juices and pastes

Herbal jams and jellies (*Paka, Leha, Avaleha*) are prepared with raw sugar (jaggery), ghee or honey, which are considered excellent tonics. The sugar acts as a preservative, improves the taste of the preparation and enhances its

Cold infusions (*Hima*)

A cold infusion involves steeping leaves, flowers or seeds, and is generally used for treating *Pitta* disorders. One part of herb is steeped in six parts of water and

CORIANDER-SEED INFUSION

Put three dessertspoons of seeds into a large cup and cover with cold water. Leave to infuse overnight. Strain and drink first thing in the morning. This is excellent for cooling heat and reducing *Pitta*, particularly for hot flushes during the menopause.

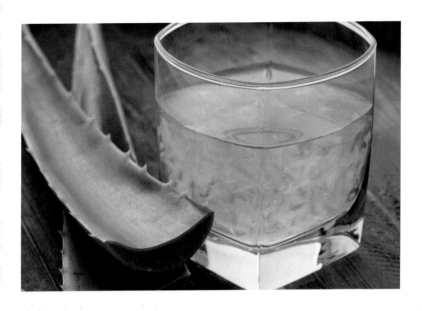

tonic properties. Jams and jellies are used as tonics for debility. Chayawanprash is the most famous of these preparations, but there are many others, including *Brahmi Rasayana* for the intellect, *Agastya Haritaki Leha* for the lungs and *Bilva Avelaha* for the intestines.

Aloe vera taken as a fresh juice is excellent for soothing inflammatory gut problems.

Chayawanprash

Ingredients: amalaki, long pepper, bamboo manna, cloves, cinnamon, cardamom, cubebs, ghee, raw sugar, sesame oil

Properties: nutritive tonic, rejuvenative. For almost any condition of weakness, or as an energy tonic for all three *doshas*, like a multivitamin and mineral supplement.

Uses: general debility, old age,

anaemia, sexual debility, coughs, convalescence, wasting, stress, lowered immunity
Dosage: 1–2 teaspoons two to three times daily in milk

Fresh juice (*Svarasa*)

The fresh juice of a plant is the best way to give juicy and aromatic plants, such as aloe vera, tulsi (*Ocimum sanctum*), ginger or brahmi (*Bacopa monniera*).

Herbal paste (*Kalka*)

Crushed fresh plants or powder mixed with water or aloe-vera gel can be made into a paste. Pastes are generally used for poultices and plasters applied externally. Vulnerary herbs that speed healing and soothe the skin include turmeric, aloe vera, neem, gotu kola and bringaraj.

Herbal wines and tinctures

There are two types of traditional herbal wines, *Asavas* and *Arishtas*. They are herbal fermentations made like grape-wine in large wooden vats. They are considered easier to digest than other herbal preparations, particularly as they contain spices, which improve not only their taste, but also their digestion and absorption. They are generally used as tonics and to stimulate the digestive fire and are particularly good for *Vata*.

Asavas are made with fresh herbal juices and *Arishtas* with decoctions of herbs – that is, they have been boiled first. Dhataki (*Woodfordia fruticosa*) flowers are added and are left to self-ferment.

Although not traditionally used in Ayurveda, tinctures are commonly employed these days in the West as a convenient way to administer herbs. Herbs are macerated in water and alcohol, generally at a ratio of one part of dried herb to five parts of liquid or one part of fresh herb to two parts of liquid. They are left for a period of at least two weeks and then pressed. These are particularly applicable for *Vata* and *Kapha*.

Kumariasava
(Aloe Herbal Wine)
Ingredients: aloe-vera gel, jaggery, honey, Trikatu, Triphala and other spices
Properties: alterative, tonic, expectorant, cooling for *Pitta*, laxative, blood tonic, liver tonic
Uses: anaemia, poor endocrine function, coughs, asthma, constipation, liver problems, chronic hepatitis
Dosage: 50–125 ml (2–4 fl oz) with meals

Arjunarishta
(Arjuna Herbal Wine)
Ingredients: arjuna, raisins, madhuka flower, dhataki, jaggery
Properties: heart tonic, cardiostimulant, balances all three *doshas*
Uses: cardiac and pulmonary disorders, blood pressure problems, high cholesterol. Emotional problems of all three *doshas*

Turmeric is respected for its digestive, detoxifying, antioxidant and anti-inflammatory properties.

Dosage: 50–125 ml (2–4 fl oz) with meals

Ashokarishta
(Ashoka Herbal Wine)
Ingredients: ashoka, dhataki, jaggery, cumin, Triphala, ginger, sandalwood
Properties: alterative, astringent, haemostatic
Uses: heavy, painful periods, blood in the urine, vaginal discharges
Dosage: 50–125 ml (2–4 fl oz) with meals

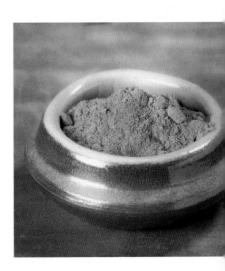

Ashwagandharishta
(Ashwagandha Herbal Wine)
Ingredients: ashwagandha, white musali, madder, liquorice, turmeric, Trikatu, sandalwood, calamus, dhataki, jaggery
Properties: nerve tonic, sedative, nourishing tonic. Calms *Vata*
Uses: nervous debility, stress, loss of memory, exhaustion, insomnia, lowered immunity, *Vata* problems
Dosage: 50–125 ml (2–4 fl oz) with meals

Draksharishta
(Grape Herbal Wine)
Ingredients: raisins and spices
Properties: stimulant, diuretic, carminative, iron tonic. Reduces *Pitta* and *Vata*.
Uses: poor appetite, indigestion, debility, insomnia, coughs; good for *Vata*-type digestive problems
Dosage: 50–125 ml (2–4 fl oz) with meals

Gugguls
Gugguls are pills made with the purified resin of the herb guggulu (*Commiphora mukul*), a relative of myrrh and a major detoxifying herb, especially good for *Vata*. Gugguls are purified by boiling them with various herbal decoctions, such as Triphala, and straining out the purified resin.

A variety of different herbal powders or extracts are added to the purified guggul resin, often with ghee. For example, *Kaishore Guggulu* is an anti-inflammatory and it is 'triturated' in aloe-vera gel. (Trituration grinds herbs by rubbing and pounding them into fine particles that are easy to digest. Friction also helps remove natural and chemical impurities.) This ground paste is then baked in an oven, ground to a powder and made into pills.

Gugguls are used for treating arthritis, nervous disorders, skin problems, high cholesterol and triglycerides and obesity.

Gokshuradi Guggulu
Ingredients: guggulu, gokshura, Trikatu, musta

Properties: diuretic, alterative, demulcent
Uses: difficult urination, urinary stones, arthritis and prostate problems
Dosage: 2–5 pills two to three times daily in cyperus tea or vetiver tea

Triphala Guggulu

Ingredients: guggulu, Triphala, long pepper
Properties: alterative, anti-inflammatory, antibiotic, antiseptic
Uses: boils, abscesses, ulcers, haemorrhoids, nasal polyps, oedema, arthritis. Cleansing and detoxifying for *Vata*, particularly in *Sama* conditions or when *Vata* has entered the lymph or blood.
Dosage: 2–5 pills two to three times daily

Kanchanar Guggulu

Ingredients: guggulu, kanchanara, Triphala, Trikatu, cardamom, cinnamon, *Crataeva religiosa*
Properties: alterative, anti-

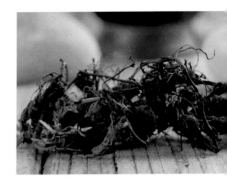

Musta root clears heat and toxins from the body and balances all three doshas.

inflammatory, lymphatic cleanser, anti-tumour, diuretic, reduces cholesterol, decongestant, thyroid regulator. Raises *Agni*, clears *Ama*, reduces *Kapha*.
Uses: tumours such as fibroids, cysts, polycystic ovarian disease, endometriosis, swollen glands, high cholesterol, low thyroid function, obesity, skin problems
Dosage: 2–5 pills two to three times daily

Kaishore Guggulu

Ingredients: guggulu, Triphala, guduchi, ginger, black pepper, pippali, *Operculina turpethum, Croton tiglium*

Properties: alterative, anti-inflammatory, diuretic, anti-arthritic, febrifuge, laxative; clears *Ama* and *Pitta*

Uses: inflammatory arthritis, gout, polymyalgia, muscle pain, inflammatory skin problems, tumours, urinary-tract infections, constipation

Dosage: 2–5 pills two to three times daily

Punarnava Guggulu

Ingredients: guggulu, punarnava, castor oil, ginger, guduchi, black pepper, pippali, Triphala, psyllium, rock salt, *Baliospermum montanum, Operculina turpethum, Semecarpus anacardium*, Swarna makshik

Properties: diuretic, alterative, demulcent

Uses: fluid retention, *Kapha*-type arthritis, gout, sciatica, urinary problems, enlargement of the prostate, obesity, diabetes, congestive heart failure

Dosage: 2–5 pills two to three times daily

Medicated ghees and oils

Medicated ghees (*Siddha ghrta*) are used to nourish the nerves and mind. As ghee (clarified butter) is

---

SHATAVARI GHEE

100 gm (3½ oz) shatavari

800 ml (28 fl oz) water

400 ml (14 fl oz) ghee

Simmer the shatavari and water down to 200 ml (7 fl oz) decoction. Then add to the ghee and simmer until the water has evaporated and it is a sludgy consistency, like ghee.

easily absorbed into the deeper tissues, it makes a good vehicle to carry herbs into the body. Being nourishing and cooling, medicated ghee is generally used for *Vata* and *Pitta* diseases.

One part of herb is heated in four parts of ghee and 16 parts of water until the water evaporates. *Brahmi ghrta* and *Panchtikta ghrta* are renowned ghee compounds.

Medicated oils

Medicated oils (*Siddha taila*) combine many different tonic herbs, generally in sesame oil, and are used in massage and oil therapy for external nourishment. Made the same way as ghee (one part herb to four parts oil and 16 of water), these decocted oils are used for pain, inflammation, arthritis, tense and aching muscles, neuralgia, trauma, healing wounds, strengthening bones, and as hair tonics, skin treatments, medicated enemas and vaginal douches. They are also used for nasal administration (*Nasya*) to clear catarrhal congestion and sinus conditions. They can be taken internally, such as when Mahanaryan oil is used to clear asthma.

Bringaraj Taila
(Eclipta Oil)
Ingredients: bringaraj juice, sesame oil
Properties: antiseptic, hair tonic, nervine, anti-inflammatory for the skin
Uses: premature greying/balding, alopecia, itching inflamed skin and scalp. An excellent hair and scalp conditioner. Also calms the mind.

Brahmi Taila
(Gotu Kola Oil)
Ingredients: gotu kola, bacopa and other nervine herbs in coconut oil
Properties: nervine, sedative, antipyretic, vulnerary, anti-inflammatory
Uses: insomnia, mental agitation, headache, eye pain, premature greying/balding, skin problems,

HERBAL VEHICLES

Herbal remedies are prepared in different carriers according to the predominant *dosha* being treated. These carriers are known as *Anupana* or herbal vehicles, and act to augment or modify the action of the herb with which they are mixed. Milk, water, ghee, oil, herb juices, sugar, salt and honey are all used as vehicles.

• **Milk** counteracts *Pitta* and *Vata* and also enhances the nourishing effect of tonics such as ashwagandha (*Withania somnifera*) or shatavari (*Asparagus racemosus*)

• **Water,** when hot, increases *Agni*, clears *Ama* and reduces *Vata* and *Kapha*; when cool, it reduces *Pitta*

• **Ghee** carries the herbs deep into the tissues, nourishes the nervous and reproductive systems and improves the digestion and absorption of the remedy; it is particularly useful for *Pitta*

• **Honey** clears *Kapha* due to its warming astringency

cuts and wounds. It is a general brain tonic.

Mahanaryan Taila
(Mahanaryan Oil)
Ingredients (main ones; it contains 58 herbs): shatavari, cow's milk, ashwagandha, castor root, gokshura, neem, bilva, bala, sesame oil
Properties: demulcent, emollient, analgesic, anti-inflammatory
Uses: arthritis, gout, muscle tension and pain, nerve pain, paralysis. It is the most commonly used oil for arthritis.

Chapter 17: *Panchakarma*

Panchakarma is deep and thorough cleansing of the *srotas*. It requires proper guidance from a highly trained Ayurvedic practitioner, so it necessitates in-patient care in special therapy centres. There are some existing centres in the UK, USA and Europe, but otherwise this treatment is plentiful in India and Sri Lanka. A specific *Panchakarma* programme is devised with each individual's constitution, disorders or needs in mind and requires close observation and supervision.

Panch means 'five' and *karma* means 'actions' as *Panchakarma* comprises five types of treatment for clearing excess *doshas* and removing toxins. These practices are extremely helpful in relieving deep-seated diseases, as well as for maintaining and improving physical and mental health:

1 *Vamana* (vomiting)
2 *Virechana* (purgation)
3 *Basti* (enema or colonic irrigation)
4 *Nasya* (nose-cleaning)
5 *Raktamokshana* (blood-cleansing)

Shirodhara *involves pouring warm oil on the forehead for 30 to 40 minutes and is a wonderful remedy for calming* Vata.

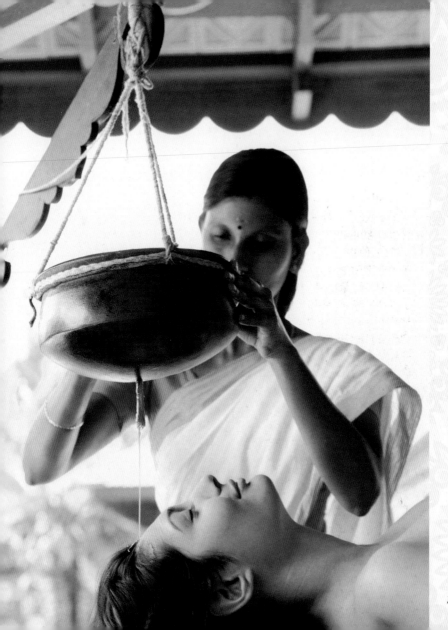

The three phases

There are actually three integrated components of the *Panchakarma* process: the preparation phase, the principal procedures and the post-procedure phase, as described below.

Preparation phase (*Purvakarma*)

Purvakarma treatments are designed to relax body and mind, improve the flow of energy by opening the *srotas* (channels) and prepare the body to eliminate toxins. They include light fasting, *Snehana* (massaging the body with herbal oils) and taking herbal decoctions or oils followed by *Swedana* (steam therapy). They help loosen accumulated toxins (*Ama*), which then enter the major channels of the body for elimination.

After 4–14 days of *Purvakarma* the *doshas* have usually settled in their sites of origin in the gastrointestinal tract, and *Ama* is ready to be flushed from the system by the appropriate *Panchakarma* treatment.

Internal *Purvakarma* involves taking medicated ghee preparations in increasing quantities for two to six days, usually before external oil therapy.

External *Purvakarma* involves:
• **Snehana**: Oil is massaged into the entire body (using two- or four-handed *Abhyanga*, *Shirodhara*, and so on) and can be very relaxing, helping to reduce stress and nourish the nervous system. Oil massage helps facilitate the removal of accumulated *Ama*. The body is massaged daily for three to seven days for 45–60 minutes, with strokes that encourage the

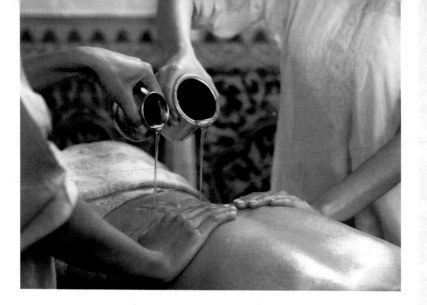

movement of toxins toward the
gastrointestinal tract.

*Oil massage is not only relaxing but
also helps facilitate the removal of
accumulated toxins.*

• *Swedana*: This is the therapeutic
application of steam to cause
sweating and is recommended
immediately following oil massage.
It is designed to dilate the *srotas,*
liquefy and remove impurities
through the skin and
gastrointestinal tract, and is
accelerated by the addition of
herbal preparations. After *Swedana*
a herbal powder such as
sandalwood, rose or vacha powder

is often rubbed on the skin, which
helps the circulation, removes
toxins and calms imbalanced *doshas*.
Afterwards you shower and rest.

After three to seven days of
Snehana and *Swedana* the *doshas*
become well 'ripened'. The correct
Panchakarma method is then
administered, according to your
constitution (*Prakruti*) and your
disorder (*Vikruti*) respectively.

Principal procedures (Pradhanakarma)

As mentioned on page 360, there are five basic types of treatment during this phase of *Panchakarma*.

1 *Vamana* (therapeutic vomiting)

Vamana is the use of emetics to clear excess *Kapha* and accumulated toxins. Daily treatment involves loosening and mobilizing the toxins to enable them to be eliminated more easily. For one to three days prior to *Vamana* you follow a *Kapha*-increasing diet, and generally drink a cup of recommended oil two or three times a day until the stool becomes oily or you feel nauseous. Oil massage and steam are recommended on the night before doing *Vamana*.

First thing in the morning, during *Kapha* time, you take three or four glasses of liquorice or salt water, then stimulate vomiting by rubbing the tongue, which triggers the gag reflex. This can often release repressed emotions that

> ### CONTRAINDICATIONS FOR *VAMANA*
>
> Avoid below the age of 12 or over 65; one week before and during menstruation; during pregnancy, high *Vata* and the *Vata* season; in emaciation, acute fear, grief or anxiety, hypoglycaemia, heart disease, acute fever and diarrhoea.

have been held in the *Kapha* areas of the lungs and stomach, along with the accumulated *dosha*. *Kapha* symptoms such as congestion, wheezing and breathlessness can disappear very quickly. Afterwards you generally fast until 5 p.m., then eat *Kichari* (see recipe on page 215) with ghee. You can drink cumin, coriander, ginger or fennel tea, or hot water with fresh lime juice with a teaspoon of honey.

Therapeutic vomiting is indicated in chronic asthma, diabetes, lymphatic congestion, chronic indigestion, oedema, bronchitis, colds, coughs, chronic allergies, hay fever, vitiligo, psoriasis, hyperacidity, chronic nasal congestion, obesity, psychological disorders and skin problems.

2 *Virechana* (purgation)

Virechana is the use of herbal purgatives, including senna leaves, prunes, bran, flaxseed husk, psyllium seed, castor oil, raisins, mango juice and Triphala, in individually tailored combinations. It is intended to remove *Pitta* toxins that accumulate in the liver, gall bladder and gastrointestinal tract and cause symptoms such as skin rashes and inflammation, acne, nausea and jaundice. Purgation should be used together with the correct diet for the predominant *dosha*. Although senna-leaf tea is a mild laxative, it can cause people with a high *Vata* constitution to have griping pain. An effective laxative for *Vata* or *Pitta* constitutions is a glass of hot milk with two teaspoons of ghee, taken at night.

Purgation is indicated in chronic fevers, diabetes, asthma, skin disorders such as herpes, vitiligo, psoriasis, allergic rashes and inflammation, acne, eczema, digestive disorders, hyperacidity, headaches, gynaecological disorders, liver problems, jaundice, urinary disorders, worms and parasites, burning sensations and inflammation of the eyes, conjunctivitis and joint disorders, including gout.

3 *Basti* (enema or colonic irrigation)

Basti using medicated oil or ghee and herbal decoctions is considered the most important *Panchakarma* treatment because it clears accumulated toxins from all three *doshas* through the bowel, and is highly beneficial as a rejuvenating treatment. It is particularly indicated in all *Vata* problems, and *Vata* is the main causative factor in

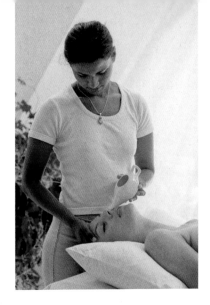

Nasya *is excellent for clearing accumulated toxins from the head that block the flow of* Prana.

CONTRAINDICATIONS FOR *BASTI*

Diarrhoea, rectal bleeding, chronic indigestion; fevers, breathlessness, diabetes, emaciation, severe anaemia, pulmonary tuberculosis; old age and children under seven.

the manifestation of all diseases. The principal site of *Vata* is the bowel, but bone tissue (*Asthi dhatu*) is another important site, so enemas are especially helpful for bone and joint problems. Enemas are generally given daily for 8–30 days, depending on the medical condition of the patient.

Enemas are indicated in nervous disorders, colitis, convalescence, poor circulation, irritable bowel syndrome, constipation, wind, bloating, digestive disorders, obesity, piles, sexual debility, infertility, kidney stones, cervical spondylosis, arthritis, gout, muscle spasms, backache and sciatica, and headaches. Hemiplegia (paralysis of one side of the body) and paraplegia are also treated with enemas.

4 *Nasya* (nasal administration)

Nasya involves administration of medicated oil through the nose, to help clear accumulated toxins from the head and neck region. It is generally given for up to 30 days, depending on the patient's medical condition. The nose is the gateway to the brain and thus to consciousness. *Prana*, the life force, enters the body through the breath. It travels to the brain and maintains sensory and motor functions, mental activities such as memory, concentration and the intellect. Deranged *Prana* disturbs the mind and can lead to symptoms such as headaches, convulsions, loss of memory and reduced sensory perception.

Substances used in *Nasya* include brahmi, ginger, ghee, oils, decoctions, vacha, long pepper, black pepper, rose and jasmine.

Nasya is indicated in trigeminal neuralgia, poor memory and eyesight, insomnia, excess mucus, hyperpigmentation in the face, premature greying of hair, headaches, loss of smell and taste, frozen shoulder, migraine, stiff neck, nasal allergies and polyps, nervous and neurological problems, Bell's palsy, hemiplegia, paraplegia and sinusitis.

5 *Raktamokshana* (blood-cleansing)

Raktamokshana involves extracting a small amount of blood from a vein to relieve tension caused by excess *Pitta*. *Pitta* is produced from disintegrated red blood cells in the liver, so *Pitta* and blood have a very close relationship. Increased *Pitta* and *Ama* may cause skin disorders such as rashes, eczema and scabies, as well as liver problems and gout.

Raktamokshana is used rarely, due to the risk of infection. However, there are blood-cleansing herbs that can be used instead, in conjunction with a *Pitta*- and *Ama*-reducing diet. Bitter and astringent foods and herbs such as saffron, guduchi, rose, turmeric, neem and pomegranate juice all help purify the blood.

Post-procedure phase

The third step, or post-detoxification, is important because this is the optimum time to take *Rasayanas* (see Chapter 18) – the Ayurvedic elixirs that rejuvenate the body and help stop

CONTRAINDICATIONS FOR *RAKTAMOKSHANA*

Anaemia, oedema, weakness; young children and old age; during pregnancy and menstruation.

ageing – such as ashwagandha and Chayawanprash.

General advice

During all *Panchakarma* treatments it is important to get plenty of rest and to avoid strenuous exercise, sex, late nights, loud music, television, over-stimulation, cold drinks and cold food, caffeine, white sugar, recreational drugs, cigarettes, alcohol and dairy products. Keep warm and away from cold and wind, and observe your thoughts and emotions during this time.

To rest the digestive fire, a diet of *Kichari* and ghee is recommended because during *Panchakarma*, when toxins move back into the

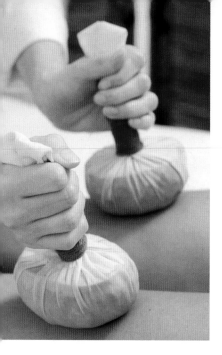

Pinda Sweda is used to massage the body and enhance sweating. It is excellent for relieving muscle and joint pain.

transitions foster accumulations of a specific *dosha*, cleansing yourself at these times can be helpful in reducing or eliminating those accumulations. At the end of a cold, dry autumn in early winter, *Vata* accumulates. At the end of a cold, wet spring, *Kapha* accumulates. By the end of a warm, humid summer, *Pitta* will have increased. These are ideal times to undergo *Panchakarma* and restore balance to the body.

Other *Panchakarma* therapies include *Shirodhara*, in which medicated water or milk and herbal oils are poured continuously on the forehead in a special method for 30–45 minutes; and *Pinda Sweda*, when a heated bolus made from grains, herbs and milk is used to firmly massage the entire body and encourage sweating, paying special attention to the joints.

gastrointestinal tract, our digestive power is reduced. *Kichari* nourishes the tissues of the body, is excellent for rejuvenation of the cells and helps the detoxification process. Basmati rice and mung dahl or lentils create a balanced meal with plenty of protein and are *tridoshic*.

A few days of *Panchakarma* are recommended at the change of seasons. Because the seasonal

Chapter 18: The concept of *Rasayana*

Rasayana, or rejuvenation therapy, is one of the eight main branches of Ayurveda and is recommended to increase *Ojas* (life force) after detoxification programmes. It is also excellent for the elderly, pregnant women, children, those who are nervously run-down, debilitated or emaciated, when convalescing, after childbirth, and for anaemia and *Vata* conditions.

Rasayana therapy is particularly good for *Vata* types during the autumn, to give them weight and strength and help them endure the long, cold winter. It is contra-indicated in any condition associated with *Ama* (toxins), for obese people, and during colds and flu, congestive disorders, fevers, infectious diseases and allergies.

For 5,000 years or so, the wisdom of Ayurveda has provided guidelines for slowing down the ageing process (*Jara*) by increasing *Ojas*. Modern scientific evaluation of *Rasayana* plants and other treatments used in Ayurveda have borne out the fact that rejuvenative tonics have the ability to protect the body against the ravages of age and the damaging effects of the environment in which we live, by enhancing the body's ability to fight off disease-carrying organisms through non-specifically activating the immune system.

The lotus is held sacred in India, where it is revered as the symbol of purity, peace, transcendence, enlightenment and rebirth.

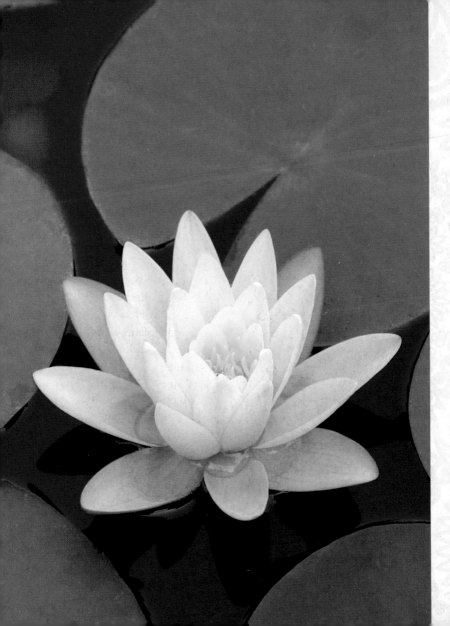

Rejuvenating body and mind

Many *Rasayana* herbs have adaptogenic properties, enhancing our resilience to stress, whether it is physical (in the shape of overwork, pollution, the use of alcohol and drugs, for example) or emotional (from grief, anxiety and so on).

Many of these herbs contain antioxidants, which help to prevent the damage caused by free radicals. According to Ayurveda, *Rasayanas* bring about proper nourishment, growth and enhanced function of all seven tissues (*dhatus*).

Rejuvenation therapy affects body and mind at the same time. It prevents the effects of early ageing on both, and increases the body's resistance to disease. According to the Ashtanga Hridarya, *Rasayana* includes nourishing the body with 'milk, raw sugar, ghee and honey, with oil enemas, by sleeping and resting freely, by oil massage, by baths and comfortable lifestyle'. In fact any herb or diet that enlivens the body and mind and enhances immunity is considered to be rejuvenative.

In *Rasayana* therapy it is recommended that excess work (physical and mental) should be reduced; you should go to bed early, sleep as much as you desire, reduce sexual activity, avoid stimulation from mass-media entertainment, practise *Pranayama* (breathing exercises) and gentle exercise like yoga or qi'gong to build energy, and spend time in nature, such as by the sea, in a mountain cabin or in a beautiful and peaceful place.

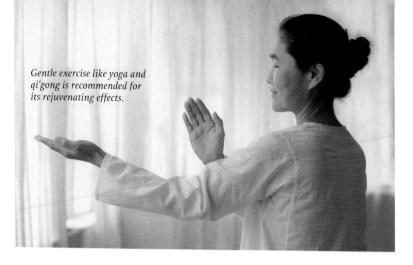

Gentle exercise like yoga and qi'gong is recommended for its rejuvenating effects.

Ojas

The substance known as *Ojas* is central to rejuvenation. It is said to be the eighth tissue, or the essence of all the body tissues. It is the ultimate product of digestion and the nutrition of all seven *dhatus*, as well as the prime energy reserve of the entire body. It provides the vitality, bodily strength, 'get up and go' and *joie de vivre* that get us through life. It is the subtle essence of all *Kapha* in the body, and specifically the essence of the reproductive fluid. *Ojas* reflects the condition or excellence of the body as a whole. Our immunity, fertility, longevity, strength and resistance depend on the quality and quantity of *Ojas*. Illness and loss of immunity arise from *Ojas* depletion. All rejuvenation therapies are therefore targeted at improving our *Ojas*.

Rejuvenating foods

Tonic foods and herbs that nurture *Ojas* tend to be heavy and nourishing, and can be hard to digest, so the state of *Agni* (digestive fire) needs to be considered first. Tonifying foods are similar to those that calm *Vata*, but the diet can be modified according to the balance of *doshas* in each individual.

- *Kichari* (see page 215) is one of the best basic foods for tonification, and can often be digested when nothing else can.

- Dairy produce is good for debility and convalescence and is considered to strengthen *Ojas*. Ghee is said to be the best food for restoring vitality, nourishing the nerves and increasing *Ojas*.

- Nuts and seeds strengthen the nerves, improve vitality and are excellent meat substitutes. Nut butters are good. Also walnuts, pine nuts, coconut, black sesame seeds and lotus seeds.

- Grains are strengthening, although not as much as nuts and seeds. Wheat, oats and brown rice are said to be best.

- Beans are good meat substitutes, but hard to digest for *Vata*, so they are better for *Pitta* and *Kapha*. Black gram, chickpeas, mung beans and tofu are best.

- Most fruit and vegetables are too light to provide strength, but sweeter-tasting ones can improve vitality and help rebuild tissues – for instance, dates, raisins, figs, pomegranates, black grapes, okra, potatoes, sweet potatoes, yams and onions cooked in ghee.

- Garlic, ginger, cinnamon and long pepper are warming and strengthening and can improve energy, especially when combined with oils such as ghee. They help to maintain good digestive fire. Black pepper, cardamom, cloves, fennel, cumin, coriander, asafoetida and a little cayenne are useful cooked in ghee with other tonic foods.

- Raw sugar gives strength and helps to build body tissues. Jaggery (pure cane sugar) is best, as it is rich in minerals and

---

RASAYANA OILS

- For *Vata*: Angelica, calamus, aloe vera, Himalayan cedarwood, frankincense, geranium, ginger, gotu kola, jasmine, jatamansi, lotus, myrrh, rose, saffron, sandalwood and vetiver
- For *Pitta*: Aloe vera, Himalayan cedarwood, gotu kola, jasmine, lotus and saffron
- For *Kapha*: Aloe vera, angelica, calamus, Himalayan cedarwood, frankincense, jasmine, lotus, myrrh, rose and saffron

---

easiest to digest. Also good are honey, raw sugar, maple syrup, rock candy, molasses, malt sugar, lactose and fructose.

- Adequate salt intake is part of a tonifying diet.

Essential oils

Rasayana oils have properties that go beyond the realm of physical healing. They are capable of healing deep emotions and improve the harmony of the mind. Vasant Lad, one of the foremost experts on Ayurvedic medicine, says they contain a spiritual energy that helps free us from attachment to the physical world and enable a deep connection with the divine and oneness.

Behavioural rejuvenation

There are many activities that promote health and happiness, known as behavioural *Rasayanas* (*Achara Rasayanas*). They

RASAYANA HERBS

The world of herbs is replete with amazing plants that nourish us, increase our physical strength and stamina and enhance our immunity. As such, they can enliven both mind and body and help counter the effects of ageing. They include: gotu kola, shatavari, bacopa, amalaki, pippali, bala, guduchi, ashwagandha, turmeric, tulsi, aloe vera, vidari, gokshura and the formula Triphala.

strengthen our life force by stimulating positive emotions and experiences, which promote the production of *Ojas*. Uplifting emotions and a positive approach to life are qualities that can be engendered over time. The most important trigger is the regular experience of our inner life, the Self or pure consciousness. Ayurvedic texts mention a number of behavioural *Rasayanas*:

• Encourage positive emotions and experiences, and do not give too much space to negative emotions. Pure joy is the best recipe for eliminating mental *Ama*.

• Choose to be with wise people, who inspire you to strive for greater knowledge, wisdom, love and consideration of others, compassion and charity.

• Be truthful, but always speak the truth with kindness.

• Maintain your personal integrity, which enhances your self-esteem.

• Maintain cleanliness in all things: mental, physical and environmental. A clean and beautiful environment will uplift you, engendering positive emotions and a sense of well-being that is health-inducing.

• Be charitable and generous. Give money, knowledge, advice and encouragement to others.

• Follow your own spiritual beliefs, devoting time to spiritual practices that provide a channel enabling love to flow.

• Sit quietly and watch the breath, or choose your own kind of meditation or contemplation.

• Do what you love to do and experience pure joy, without hurting anyone else – for instance, by painting or watching nature.

• Cook for your family with love and respect. If you are eating out, say prayers over your food to remove any negativity.

• Observe silence, for it is very nourishing.

Maintaining cleanliness is considered important to living a long life.

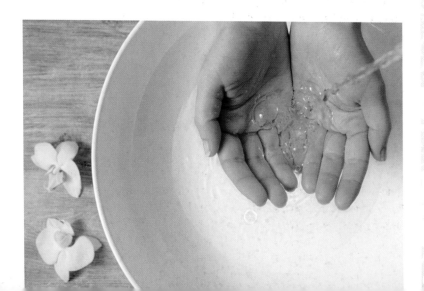

Glossary of Sanskrit terms

Abhyanga: warm oil massage

Agni: digestive fire/enzymes

Ahamkara: ego, or the sense of 'I-ness'

Ahararasa: the nutrient chyle

Akasha: ether/space

Alochaka Pitta: one of the five subtypes of **Pitta**, governing vision

Ama: toxins/the undigested food mass

Amla: sour, one of the six **Rasas** or tastes

Anupana: vehicle (such as honey) to carry herbs to the tissues

Apana Vata: one of the five subtypes of Vata, governing the elimination of waste energy and relating to the colon and lower abdomen

Arishta: herbal wine made with decoctions

Artha: prosperity, one of the four goals in life

Asana: yoga posture

Asava: herbal wine made with the juice of herbs

Asthi: bone tissue

Atman: inner or higher self

Avalambaka Kapha: the main of five subtypes of **Kapha**, governing the heart and lungs

Bala tantra: gynaecology, obstetrics and paediatrics

Basti: enema, one of the five *Panchakarma* therapies

Bhutagnis: five digestive enzymes that metabolize the five elements

Bhuta vidya: psychiatry, the treatment of mental disease

Bodhaka Kapha: one of the five subtypes of *Kapha*, governing taste

Brahma: the Absolute reality, pure consciousness

Brajaka Pitta: one of the five subtypes of *Pitta*, governing complexion

Brimhana: tonifying therapy

Buddhi: inner wisdom within the individual

Chayawanprash: herbal rejuvenative jam

Chikitsa: Ayurvedic treatment

Chitta: the storehouse of our experiences

Churna: herbal powder

Dharma: career, life purpose or path, one of the four goals in life

Dhatuagnis: seven digestive enzymes that metabolize the seven tissues

Dhatus: tissue layers

Dinacharya: daily routine

Doshas: the biological 'humours', or life forces, that govern our constitution

Draksharishta: herbal wine made from grapes and other spices

Ghee: clarified butter

Gunas: three qualities or fundamental laws of nature

Jaggery: a form of pure cane sugar

Jala: water/cohesive factor

Jatharagni: digestive enzymes in the gastrointestinal tract/ digestive 'fire'

Jibha pariksha: tongue diagnosis

Kama: enjoyment, one of the four goals of life

Kanjee: barley-water and rice

Kapha: biological water-humour, one of the *doshas*

Karma: action and reaction, cause and effect

Kasaya: astringent, one of the six *Rasas* or tastes

Katu: pungent, one of the six *Rasas* or tastes

Kichari: basmati rice and mung beans/red lentils, taken when fasting

Kitta: waste material in food

Kledaka Kapha: one of the five subtypes of *Kapha*, governing digestion

Kvatha: herbal decoction

Langhana: reduction or lightening therapy

Lavana: salty, one of the six *Rasas* or tastes

Madhura: sweet, one of the six *Rasas* or tastes

Mahat: cosmic consciousness

Majja: marrow and nerve tissue

Malas: waste products (such as urine, sweat, faeces)

Mamsa: muscle tissue

Manas: the lower/outer mind

Marma: energy points on the body

Medas: fat tissue

Medhya: the mind, intellect

Moksha: self-realization/ liberation/spiritual enlightenment, one of the four goals in life

Mutra: urine, one of the three primary waste materials

Nadi: nerve channels

Nadi pariksha: pulse diagnosis

Nasya: nasal application of herbs and oils, one of the five *Panchakarma* therapies

Neti: a small pot (netty pot) used for nasal cleansing

Nidana: diagnosis, etiology, the cause of disease

Ojas: strength, the prime energy reserve of the body

Pachaka Pitta: the main of the five subtypes of *Pitta*, governing digestion

Panchakarma: the five purification practices of Ayurveda

Pitta: biological fire-humour, one of the *doshas*

Prakruti: our constitution or primordial nature

Prana: life force, inward-moving air

Prana Vata: the primary wind or energy in the body, one of the five subtypes of *Vata*, governing the head, mind or chest

Pranayama: breathing exercises

Prithvi: earth/mass

Purisha: faeces, one of the three primary waste materials

Purusha: pure, passive, unmanifest consciousness

Purvakarma: preparatory *Panchakarma* therapies

Rajas: the quality of energy and action, one of the three *gunas*; agitation

Rakta: blood tissue

Raktamokshana: blood-cleansing, one of the five *Panchakarma* therapies

Ranjaka Pitta: one of the five subtypes of *Pitta*, colouring the blood

Rasa: plasma, one of the seven tissues/tastes before digestion

Rasayana: rejuvenation therapy and tonics

Roga: disease

Rukshana: drying therapy

Sadhaka Pitta: one of the five subtypes of *Pitta*, governing the heart and brain

Sama: *Ama* condition associated with one of the three *doshas*

Sama Kapha: *Ama* condition of *Kapha*

Sama Pitta: *Ama* condition of *Pitta*

Sama Vata: *Ama* condition of *Vata*

Samana Vata: one of the subtypes of *Vata*, governing digestion and relating to the stomach and small intestine

Samprapti: the course of disease

Sankhya: the system of enumerology; one of the six

classical schools of Indian philosophy

Sara: the pure or nutritive part of food; quality of the tissues

Sattva: the quality of clarity and harmony, one of the three *gunas*

Shamana: detoxifying palliative therapy

Shodhana: detoxifying purification therapy, or *Panchakarma*

Shukra: reproductive tissue

Sleshaka Kapha: one of the five subtypes of *Kapha*, a form of water lubricating the joints

Snehana: oil application

Srotas: the channel systems of the body

Stambhana: astringency

Sveda: sweat, one of the three primary waste materials

Swasthya: health

Swedana: therapeutic sweating, steam therapy

Taila: medicated oil, mainly using sesame oil

Tamas: the quality of decay and inertia, one of the three *gunas*

Tarpaka Kapha: one of the five subtypes of *Kapha*, in the heart and brain

Tattva: cosmic principle

Teja: fire/radiant energy

Tikta: bitter, one of the six *Rasas* or tastes

Tridosha: the three *doshas* or basic forces of the universe

Udana Vata: one of the subtypes of *Vata*, governing exhalation and relating to the throat

Unani Tibb: the Islamic system of medicine

Upadhatu: secondary tissue

Vamana: therapeutic vomiting, one of the five *Panchakarma* therapies

Vata: biological air-humour, one of the *doshas*

Vayu: air/wind, motion

Vedas: ancient scriptures of India

Vikruti: the present *doshic* imbalance of *Vata/Pitta/Kapha* in an individual

Vipaka: the post-digestive effect of a herb

Virechana: purgation, one of the five *Panchakarma* therapies

Virya: the energy of a herb, as experienced during digestion

Vyadhi: ill health or disease

Vyana Vata: one of the five subtypes of *Vata,* governing the circulation

Glossary of Western terms

Abortifacient: causes abortion

Adaptogenic: helps to restore balance within the body

Allergen: a substance that provokes an allergic response

Alterative: produces beneficial effects through detoxification

Anabolic: helps in constructive metabolic processes

Analgesic: alleviates pain without causing loss of consciousness

Anodyne: relieves pain

Anorexia: loss of appetite

Antacid: reduces stomach acid

Anthelmintic: destructive to intestinal worms

Anti-allergenic: reduces allergic reactions

Antibacterial: destroys bacteria or suppresses their growth or reproduction

Anticoagulant: retards the formation of blood clots

Anticonvulsant: prevents or relieves convulsions

Antidepressant: alleviates depression

Antidiarrhoetic: relieves diarrhoea

Anti-emetic: prevents vomiting

Antifungal: destroys fungi or suppresses their growth or reproduction

Antihaemorrhagic: stops bleeding

Antihistamine: counteracts the effects of histamine, relieving allergies

Antihypertensive: reduces high blood pressure

Anti-inflammatory: counteracts the inflammatory process

Antilithic: prevents and dissolves stones in the gall bladder, kidney and bladder

Antimalarial: effective against malaria

Antimicrobial: kills microorganisms or suppresses their multiplication or growth

Antioxidant: significantly delays or prevents oxidation and the ageing process

Antiparasitic: destroys or inhibits parasites

Antipyretic: reduces fever

Antiseptic: inhibits the growth and development of microorganisms

Antispasmodic: relieves spasm, usually of smooth muscle

Antitumour: combats the formation of tumours

Antitussive: helps to stop coughing

Antiviral: destroys viruses or suppresses their replication

Aphrodisiac: stimulates sexual desire

Astringent: causes contraction, drying

Auto-immune: relating to an immune response by the body against its own cells or tissues

Bronchodilator: widens the bronchi of the lungs

Carcinogenic: cancer-causing

Cardio-tonic: has a tonic effect on the heart

Carminative: relieves flatulence and pain

Cholagogue: promotes bile flow into the duodenum

Contraindicated: suggests that a particular drug or treatment should not be used

Decoction: a herbal formulation prepared by boiling the plant parts in water

Decongestant: reduces congestion or swelling

Demulcent: a soothing, mucilaginous or oily formulation that reduces irritation of inflamed surfaces

Depurative: purifying or cleansing

Detoxification: the reduction or removal of toxins and wastes

Diaphoretic: promotes perspiration

Digestive: aids the process of digestion

Diuretic: promotes the excretion of urine

Emetic: causes vomiting

Emmenagogue: promotes menstrual flow

Emollient: softens or soothes irritated skin or mucous membranes

Expectorant: loosens phlegm and eases its expulsion from the respiratory tract

Febrifuge: reduces body temperature during fever

Free radical: a highly reactive molecule with an unpaired electron that causes damage to tissues

Galactagogue: promotes the flow of milk

Haematuria: blood in the urine

Haemostatic: checks bleeding; **styptic**

Hepatoprotective: protects the liver

Hypoglycaemic: lowers glucose in the blood

Hypotensive: lowers blood pressure

Immunomodulatory: alters immune responses

Immunoregulator: regulates immune responses

Immunostimulant: stimulates immune responses

Immunosuppressant: suppresses immune responses

Insecticidal: selectively poisonous to insects

Laxative: promotes bowel movements

Lithotriptic: dissolves urinary and gall-bladder stones

Lymphatic: relates to the lymph system

Nervine: a nerve restorative, mildly tranquillizing

Nutritive: nourishing

Parturient: a substance that facilitates childbirth

Pathogenic: disease-causing

Potentiate: to increase the power or effect of something

Probiotic: stimulates the growth of beneficial microorganisms

Purgative: stimulates vigorous bowel movements

Refrigerant: reduces bodily heat or fever

Rejuvenative: promotes feelings of youthfulness

Relaxant: reduces muscular or nervous tension and promotes relaxation

Rubefacient: reddens the skin by increasing blood flow

Sedative: allays excitement, reduces nervousness and anxiety, promotes sleep

Spermatogenic: promotes the production of sperm

Stimulant: stimulates the central nervous system

Styptic: stops bleeding, applied externally

Thermogenic: produces heat

Tonic: restores normal tone or function to tissues; boosts energy and immunity, enhances well-being

Unctuous: greasy or oily

Uterine tonic: tones the uterus and female reproductive system

Vasodilator: widens the blood vessels, lowering blood pressure

Vermifuge: expels worms or intestinal animal parasites; **anthelmintic**

Vulnerary: promotes wound-healing

Index

Acknowledgements

Picture acknowledgements

Alamy/Agencja FREE 181; /Antographer 322; /Arco Images GmbH 296, 307, 316, 337, 338; /Bon Appetit 330; /Chris Rout 183, 254; /Dinodia Photos 30, 310, 311, 328, 349; /Estelle Joeng 329; /Fancy/Marnie Burkhart 253; /Golden Hour/Balan Madhavan 298, 334; /Jochen Tack 225; /mediacolor's 223, 366; /Moment 60; /Nigel Cattlin 308; /OJO Images Ltd./Tom Merton 264; /PhotoAlto/Odilon Dimier 247; /PhotoAlto/Alix Minde 42; /Phototake Inc./Luca Tettoni 280, 340; /Robert Harding Picture Library Ltd./Luca Tettoni 158, 178; /Spice Coast Collection/Balan Madhavan 109; /Tim Hill 211; /tbkmedia.de 356; /The Art Archive/Gianni Dagli Orti 79; /ViewFinder 291; /Westend61 GmbH 369. **Corbis**/Blend Images/Jose Luis Pelaez, Inc. 373; /Historical Picture Archive 25; /In Pictures/Christopher Pillitz 203; /J. James 176; /Luca Tettoni 8; /Westend61 284. **Fotolia**/Andres Rodriguez 43; /Anna Kuznetsova 290; /Cogipix 248; /dabjola 288; /Elena Ray 1; /Elena Schweitzer 324; /emer 325; /HLPhoto 352; /istvan 292; /ittipol 300; /Jonathan Lefebvre 314; /leungchopan 317; /Only Fabrizio 319, 341; /photocrew 320; /Piotr Marcinski 154; /R_R 295; /Shariff Che'Lah 313; /Subbotina Anna 131; /Swapan 303, 306; /TheSupe87 184; /Yuri Arcurs 147. **Garden World Images**/Jenny Lily 297. **Getty Images**/Adrian Nakic 86; /Alexandra Grablewski 127; /B2M Productions 156; /Caroline von Tuempling 23; /Dex Image 151; /Dinodia Photos 233, 293; /Dougal Waters 272; /Dylan Ellis 75; /esthAlto/Frederic Cirou 36; /FoodPix/Commanding Artists/Ray Kachatorian 228; /ICHIRO 2; /Image Source 122, 377; /Imagemore Co, Ltd. 326; /India Today Group 279; /James and James 213; /James Whitaker 66; /JGI/Jamie Grill 99; /Jill Fromer 336; /Jupiterimages 81, 361; /Martine Mouchy 110; /Matthew Wakem 161, 287; /Nicholas Pitt 95; /PhotoAlto 163; /Photolibrary/AGE Fotostock/Yogesh More 318, 332; /Photolibrary/Garden World Photo/Georgianna Lane 312; /Photolibrary/Mauritius Images/CASH 173; /Photolibrary/Mauritius Images/Tomas Adel 150; /Photolibrary/Phototake/Luca Tettoni 12, 17, 192, 363; /Photolibrary/Stockbyte 243; /Robert Nickelsberg 9, 169, 343; /Ruth Jenkinson 137, 167; /Stuart O'Sullivan 239; /The Trustees of the Chester Beatty Library, Dublin 19; /Tom Le Goff 117; /Valery Rizzo 220. **Glow Images**/Imagebroker RM 4, 7, 26; /Moodboard Premium 238; /Pixtal 269; /Stockfood/Ottmar Diez 302; /Stockfood/Eising 121; /Westend61 RM 20. **Octopus Publishing Group**/Emma Neish 137; /Janine Hosegood 70, 133, 187, 207; /Mike Good 61, 232; /Russell Sadur 119, 128, 134, 145, 148, 153, 194, 197, 261, 351; /Ruth Jenkinson 54, 273; /Stephen Conroy 130, 141; /William Reavell 88. **SuperStock**/imagebroker.net 171. **Thinkstock**/Banana Stock 231; /Brand X Pictures 33; /Comstock 48; /Digital Vision/John Howard 49; /George Doyle 101, 113; /Hemera 57, 138, 251, 259, 267, 270, 371; /iStockphoto 6, 10, 29, 35, 41, 47, 125, 142, 188, 216, 218, 301, 304, 309, 344, 346, 347, 354; /Jupiterimages 68, 82, 198, 201, 204, 245, 275; /Pixland 164; /Stockbyte 65, 72, 237, 257; /ULTRA F 116, 208.

Commissioning Editor: **Liz Dean**
Managing Editor: **Clare Churly**
Deputy Art Director: **Yasia Williams-Leedham**
Designer: **Tracy Killick**
Picture Librarian: **Jennifer Veall**
Production Controller: **Susan Meldrum**